Heart Rate Management

in

Stable Angina

Heart Rate Management *in* Stable Angina

EDITED BY

Kim Fox

Professor of Clinical Cardiology
Royal Brompton Hospital
London, UK

and

Roberto Ferrari

Chief of Cardiology
University of Ferrara
Ferrara, Italy

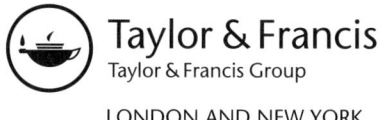

Taylor & Francis
Taylor & Francis Group

LONDON AND NEW YORK

This publication has been made possible through an educational grant from Servier. Sponsorship of this publication does not imply the sponsor's agreement or otherwise with the views expressed herein.

First published in the United Kingdom in 2005
by Taylor & Francis,
an imprint of the Taylor & Francis Group,
2 Park Square, Milton Park
Abingdon, Oxon OX14 4RN, UK

Tel.:   +44 (0) 20 7017 6000
Fax.:   +44 (0) 20 7017 6699
E-mail: info.medicine@tandf.co.uk
Website: http://www.tandf.co.uk/medicine

British Library Cataloguing in Publication Data

Data available on application

Library of Congress Cataloging-in-Publication Data

Data available on application

ISBN 1-84184-594-9

Distributed in North and South America by
Taylor & Francis
2000 NW Corporate Blvd
Boca Raton, FL 33431, USA

Within Continental USA
Tel.: 800 272 7737; Fax.: 800 374 3401
Outside Continental USA
Tel.: 561 994 0555; Fax.: 561 361 6018
E-mail: orders@crcpress.com

Distributed in the rest of the world by
Thomson Publishing Services
Cheriton House
North Way
Andover, Hampshire SP10 5BE, UK
Tel.: +44 (0) 1264 332424
E-mail: salesorder.tandf@thomsonpublishingservices.co.uk

Cover illustration: Les Laboratoires Servier.

Composition by Tracey Nichols
Printed and bound by Butler & Tanner Ltd., Frome and London, UK

Contents

Preface

Cardiovascular disease is the most important cause of morbidity and mortality worldwide; coronary heart disease makes up the majority of this burden. Patients with coronary heart disease may present with sudden death, myocardial infarction or angina pectoris. In approximately 50% of patients the initial presentation is with angina. In spite of powerful new secondary preventative treatments in patients with angina, namely aspirin, statins and ACE inhibitors, angina still remains one of the most important medical challenges affecting the western world and to an increasing extent the underdeveloped countries.

Angina occurs when myocardial oxygen demand exceeds myocardial oxygen supply causing myocardial ischemia. The most important component in terms of myocardial oxygen demand is heart rate and it has long been known that control of exercise-induced heart rate is the most important means of preventing angina. Beta-blockade has for decades been the most effective treatment for the control of angina by virtue of its action on controlling rest, and in particular, exercise heart rate. Whilst the introduction of beta-blockade revolutionized our treatment of angina, there are many patients unable to tolerate beta-blockers or still remain symptomatic in spite of treatment with them. Today we have a new pharmacological approach to the control of heart rate, namely inhibition of the I_f channels which will slow sinus node activity without affecting other components of the conduction system, (e.g. the AV node) and without having negative inotropic effects on the ventricular myocardium.

Whilst the importance of identifying new treatments that will help control the symptoms of angina cannot be underestimated, it is the equal responsibility of the physician to improve the outlook of such in terms of morbidity and mortality. It has long been known that there is a relationship between heart rate and outcome both in terms of cardiovascular mortality as well as cardiovascular morbidity, e.g. myocardial infarction and heart failure. It is therefore our hope that the introduction of a new heart-rate-slowing drug acting on the I_f channels may enlarge the armamentarium that we have already established for the secondary prevention of coronary disease and improve not only the quality of life but also life expectancy of our patients with angina.

This book provides an introduction to the most important features of angina pectoris, namely the epidemiology, pathophysiology as well as treatment. It then highlights the importance of heart rate, both in terms of morbidity and mortality and introduces us to the concept of I_f inhibition in terms of the treatment of the symptoms of angina as well as a potential indication to improve the outlook of such patients.

Kim Fox
Roberto Ferrari

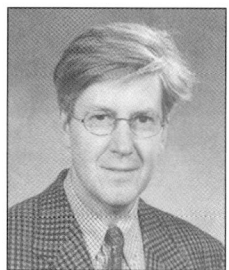

Jaap W Deckers

1 Epidemiological review of stable angina

Jaap W Deckers

Department of Cardiology
Thoraxcenter
Erasmus Medical Center
Dr Molewaterplein 40
3015 GD Rotterdam
The Netherlands
Tel:+31 10 463 5356
Email: j.deckers@erasmusmc.nl

INTRODUCTION

Chronic stable angina is the most common symptomatic manifestation of ischemic heart disease, and affects millions of men and women worldwide. The symptoms of angina are caused by a failure of sufficient oxygen to reach the heart muscle. The pathophysiologic substrate for this is almost invariably atheromatous narrowing of the coronary arteries, although others factors, such as aortic valve disease and hypertrophic cardiomyopathy, may be implicated in some patients.

The anginal episode is typically minutes in duration, and the discomfort is usually retrosternal in location, but patients may also experience radiation of pain to the neck, jaw, epigastrium, or arms.[1] Angina is commonly triggered by exertion, eating, and/or stress, and is subsequently relieved with rest. In stable angina, the frequency or severity of the activity required to trigger an attack have usually remained predictable over a prolonged period of time.[1] The severity of angina and the adverse impact that such attacks pose on the ability to carry out normal activities are predictive risk factors for subsequent ischemic complications.[2] In the Framingham study, in which 5209 initially well men and women were studied for the development of coronary heart disease (CHD), a history of CHD almost tripled the risk of a stroke.[3,4]

In US patients who have developed ischemic heart disease, stable chronic angina is the presenting symptom in approximately 50%,[5,6] and occurs in 20% of patients who subsequently experience a coronary attack.[7]

NATURAL HISTORY OF CHRONIC STABLE ANGINA

The incidence and prevalence of stable angina vary according to the population studied and the method of assessment. For instance, self-reporting by questionnaire gives higher prevalence figures than the more conservative figures obtained by physician assessment or other diagnostic testing.

By a conservative estimate, chest pain is reported by 6 800 000 Americans, with 400 000 new diagnoses of stable angina made annually.[7] Overall, significantly more women than men have stable angina.[7] However, rates are higher in men than women under the age of 70 years. This may be partly due to the protective effects of estrogens. In the US, the annual rates of new and recurrent episodes of angina per 1000 non-black men are 44.3 for the age group 65 to 74 years, 56.4 for the age group 75 to 84 years and 42.6 for the age group 85 years and older.[7] For non-black women in the same age groups, the rates are 18.8, 30.8 and 19.8, respectively. For black men, the rates are 26.1, 52.2 and 43.5, and for black women the rates are 29.4, 37.7 and 15.2, respectively.[7]

In the UK, the annual incidence of angina is estimated at 1.1 cases per 1000 males and 0.5 cases per 1000 females aged 31–70 years.[8,9] In Sweden, chest pain of ischemic origin is thought to affect 5% of all males aged 50 to 57 years.[9,10] In industrialized countries, the annual incidence of unstable angina is approximately 6 cases per 10 000 people.[9]

RELATIONSHIP WITH RISK FACTORS

Modification of lifestyle and behavioral factors, particularly smoking, diet, and exercise habits, can reduce the risk of other clinical manifestations of CHD in patients with stable chronic angina. US statistics indicate that smokers have a 70% increased risk of fatal CHD, and a 2- to 4-fold higher risk of non-fatal CHD. Cessation of smoking rapidly reduces the risk of cardiovascular events.[11,12]

Physical inactivity is also a well-recognized factor that increases the risk of cardiovascular events, and is linked to obesity. General and central obesity (measured using height, weight, skin folds, and waist girth) each make independent contributions to CHD, but central obesity is a better predictor in males.[13] Body mass index (BMI) alone is not sufficient to identify cardiovascular risk, which requires assessment of non-weight-related factors.[14] Assessment of body mass composition or waist-to-hip ratio may be more useful indicators of overweight and obesity for cardiovascular risk assessment than BMI,[15,16] most notably in lightly framed individuals.

Low physical activity level, high carbohydrate intake, and current smoking habits are also all significantly associated with an increased risk of having the metabolic syndrome.[17] The prevalence of this syndrome is increasing owing to such lifestyle habits and consequent obesity. Metabolic syndrome is attributable to a complex association of several interrelated abnormalities, the most prominent of which is insulin resistance, which increase the risk of cardiovascular disease and progression to diabetes mellitus. Metabolic syndrome is diagnosed if three or more of the following factors are present: waist circumference greater than 102 cm (40 inches) in men and 88 cm (35 inches) in women; serum triglyceride level of 150 mg/dL or higher; high-density lipoprotein (HDL) cholesterol level less than 40 mg/dL in men and 50 mg/dL in women; blood pressure of 130/85 mmHg or higher; and fasting glucose level of 110 mg/dL or higher.

Stable angina is associated with a large number of functional, atherogenic, and thrombogenic prognostic factors, including atherosclerosis and increased carotid artery intima-media thickness. In addition, evidence of coronary arterial calcification (detected by electron beam and helical-computed tomography) increases the risk of stable angina and ischemic heart disease. Other adverse factors include the presence of elevated and increasing levels of the inflammatory biomarker, C-reactive protein, which can predict future cardiovascular events independently of the severity of existing CHD.[18–20]

The epidemiological association between elevated serum cholesterol and an increased risk of ischemic heart disease has been demonstrated in numerous studies. Cholesterol lowering using statins in patients with above-average cholesterol levels has been shown to reduce the progression of atherosclerosis and lower the risk of CHD events.[21] In addition, beneficial effects of cholesterol lowering have been extended to patients with average or below-average cholesterol levels.[22,23] In men, the serum concentration of total cholesterol is the single most important blood lipid risk factor for ischemic heart disease, with high-density lipid cholesterol concentrations having a lesser role.[24] Triglyceride concentrations do not have predictive importance once other risk factors have been taken into account.[24]

Therapeutic guidelines for the management of serum cholesterol were issued by the US National Cholesterol Education Program in 2001. Subsequent clinical studies have validated the recommended targets of these guidelines.[25] The target levels for low-density lipoprotein cholesterol are < 100 to < 130 mg/dL, depending on risks; in patients considered to be at high risk, including those whose baseline levels are around 100 g/dL, it may be appropriate to reach a target level of ≤70 mg/dL as a therapeutic option. Individuals with diabetes mellitus should be considered to be within the high-risk category, due to their increased risk of CHD.[26] Men with diabetes have a cardiovascular disease risk intermediate between that of men with angina and men with previous myocardial infarction (MI).[27]

TRENDS IN CARDIOVASCULAR DISEASE

In general, during the last 20 to 30 years, improvements have been reported in mortality rates from CHD in the Western world. In New Zealand, the decline in mortality from CHD observed in males during the period 1982–1993 has been a consequence of changes in behavioral factors and the development of appropriate treatments;[28] 54% of the observed improvement was calculated to be due to lifestyle changes, and 46% due to treatments, of which treatment aimed at controlling angina contributed 9%.[28] Similarly, data from Scotland, covering almost 20 years (1975–1994), indicated that a reduction in measurable risk factors contributed to 51% of the observed reduction in mortality, while treatment contributed 41%. In Sweden, over the period 1986–1994, the prevalence of angina pectoris in the middle-aged population remained largely unchanged in men but declined slightly in women, concurrent with a decline in the proportion of individuals with high cholesterol levels.[29]

In the US, during the period 1953–1973, the 10-year mortality rate for CHD remained largely constant for men but decreased slightly for women;[30] however, the prevalence increased in both men and women. In addition, further US data from a long-term epidemiological study carried out from 1950 to 1982 showed that mortality began to decline in the 1960s but, by 1982, changing patterns of MI, as the initial manifestation of CHD, resulted in a decrease in male mortality but an increase in female mortality.[5] On the other hand, in Australia, death rates from ischemic heart disease have decreased rapidly in both men and women during the past three decades (*Figures 1 and 2*).[31]

Despite these general improvements in incidence, CHD remains a considerable cause of mortality, and its prevalence is increasing with the increasing age of western populations. This increase has led to a search for additional risk factors and additional treatments

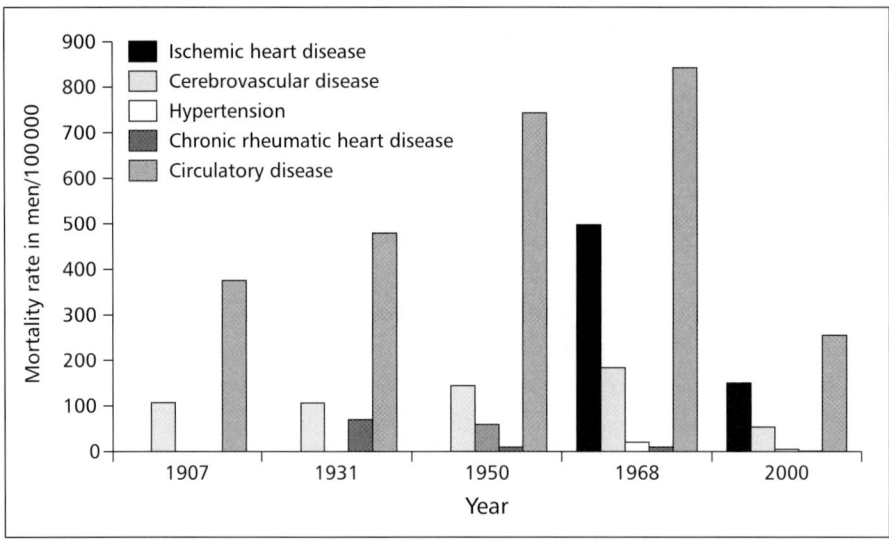

Figure 1 Trends in cardiovascular disease mortality in men, Australia (per 100 000) from 1907 to 2000

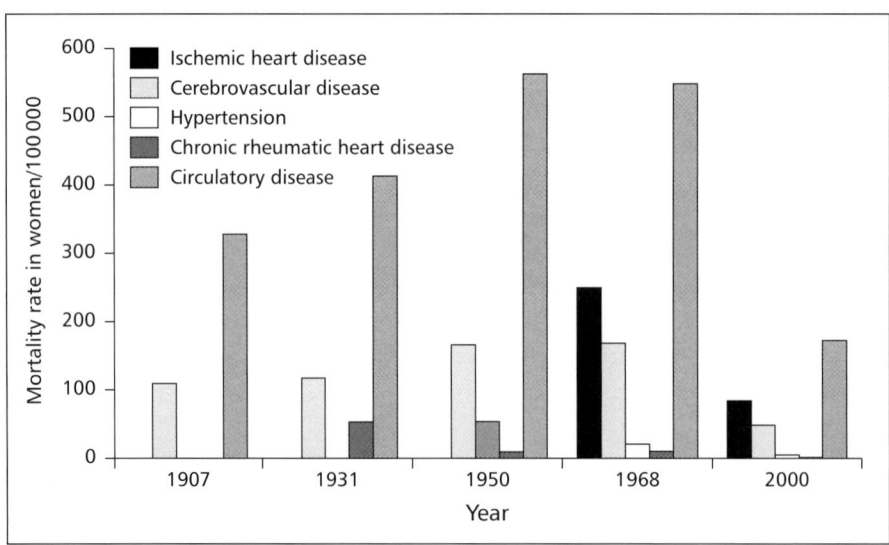

Figure 2 Trends in cardiovascular disease mortality in women, Australia (per 100 000) from 1907 to 2000

HEART RATE AS AN INDEPENDENT RISK FACTOR

In addition to the factors described above, resting heart rate has been identified as an independent risk factor for mortality from coronary disease.[32] It appears that survival is inversely related to heart rate.[33,34] Even in individuals with normal systolic blood pressure, those with heart rates ≥ 70 beats/minute have a higher risk of cardiovascular mortality.[35] A high heart rate can induce or aggravate myocardial ischemia and angina by increasing myocardial oxygen demand and decreasing myocardial perfusion. High heart rate is, therefore, a risk factor for cardiovascular mortality.[36] Among mammals, there is an inverse semilogarithmic relationship between heart rate and life expectancy,[37] and the importance of resting heart rate for influencing factors important in heart disease has been demonstrated by the use of animal models.

In cynomolgus macaques, naturally occurring differences in heart rate have been found to be associated with differences in plaque area. Monkeys with high heart rates ($n = 7$, 159 beats/min: $0.76 \, mm^2 \pm 0.21$ SD) have atherosclerotic lesions more than twice as extensive as those of monkeys with lower heart rate ($n = 8$, 133 beats/min: $0.31 \, mm^2 \pm 0.30$; $t = 3.01$, $P < 0.01$).[38] The differences are thought to be related to heart rate-induced differences in coronary blood flow. Similarly, in a study in which eight cynomolgus macaques received an atherogenic diet after either surgical ablation of the sinoatrial node (subsequently reducing resting heart rate) or a sham surgical procedure, coronary atherosclerosis was reduced in animals in whom the surgical procedure had reduced the resting heart rate.[39]

In humans, especially in men, a high resting heart rate has been associated with increased mortality from both non-cardiovascular and cardiovascular causes, and is independent of other risk factors.[40–44] This hypothesis is supported by a growing number of publications. These include, in particular the recently published study by Okamura and colleagues[45]. The results coincide with the results of a French study published by Benetos et al.[40] (*Figure 3*)

Resting heart rate is also a predictor of late mortality after MI,[46–49] and the major beneficial effects of β-blockers used post-MI, particularly the ability to prevent exercise ischemia, appear to be mediated by heart rate reduction.[36,48] In men, an elevated resting heart rate increases mortality from all major ischemic heart disease events (ischemic heart disease death and sudden cardiac death), particularly in individuals with pre-existing ischemic heart disease.[50] Conversely, epidemiological studies indicate that lowered heart rate is associated with decreased cardiovascular and all-cause mortality.[51] In men without pre-existing ischemic heart disease, elevated resting heart rate showed a strong positive correlation with cigarette smoking and BMI, and decreased significantly at higher levels of physical activity.[52] Resting heart rate in men, but not in women, is correlated with the levels of total cholesterol.[53] In the general population, assessed in a study of 9719 men and 9433 women aged 12 to 59 years, increased resting heart rate was positively associated with male gender and smoking, was observed to decrease with body height and physical activity, and showed a U-shaped relation to BMI.[54] In both sexes, a significant progressive increase in age-adjusted levels of total cholesterol, non-HDL cholesterol and triglycerides, and a decrease in HDL cholesterol, was observed with increasing resting heart rate.[54] However, there is positive correlation between minimal heart rate and the progression of coronary atheroma, independent of cholesterol concentration.[55]

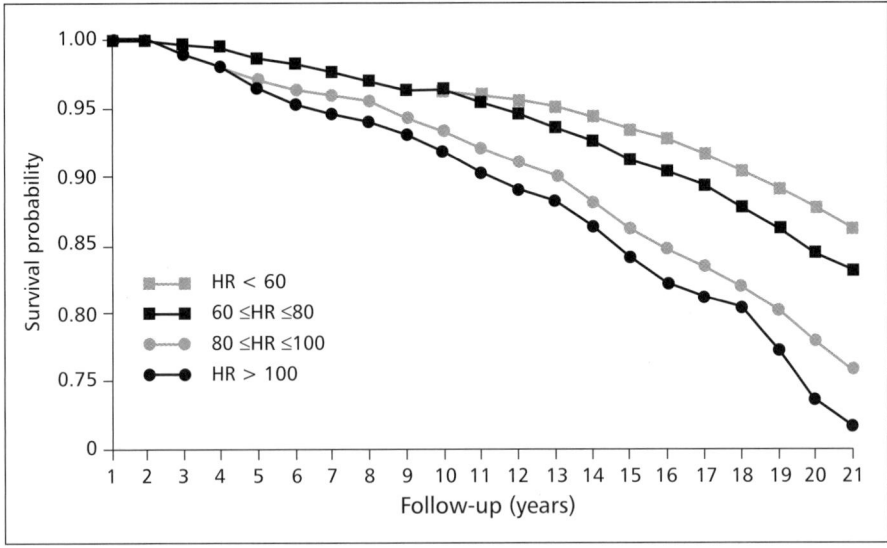

Figure 3 Survival probability curves for all cause mortality in men and women according to heart rate class. *P* values were obtained after adjustment for age, systolic blood pressure, diastolic blood pressure, cholesterol, body mass index (BMI), tobacco consumption, physical activity, antihypertensive treatment, and history of myocardial infarction[40]

The association between elevated resting heart rate and all-cause mortality is weaker in women than in men (*Figures 4–7*),[41] probably due to the diminished sympathetic tone in women compared with men.[43] However, since laboratory studies demonstrate that tachycardia may have a direct impact on the arterial wall, and can favor the occurrence of cardiac arrhythmias, high resting heart rates are also likely to be detrimental to women.[43]

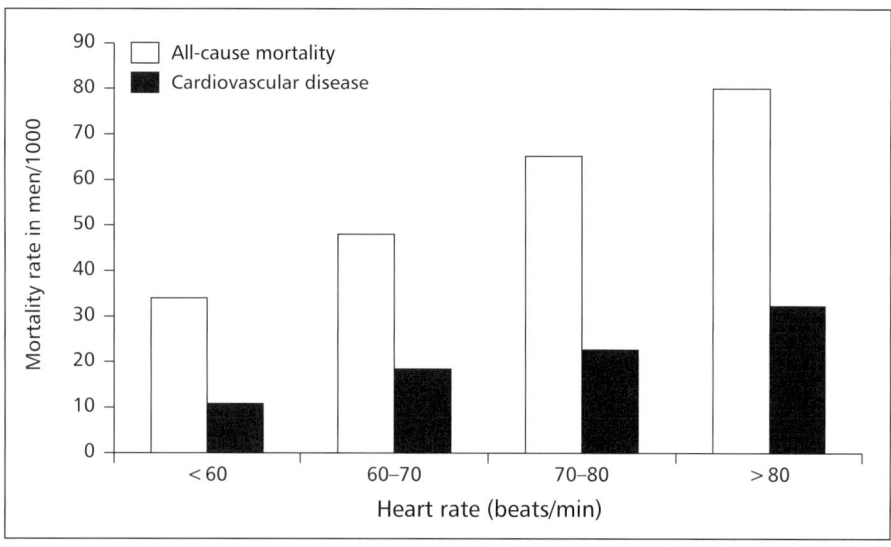

Figure 4 Mortality rate/1000 men aged 40–60 years according to initial heart rate (1982 to 1994)

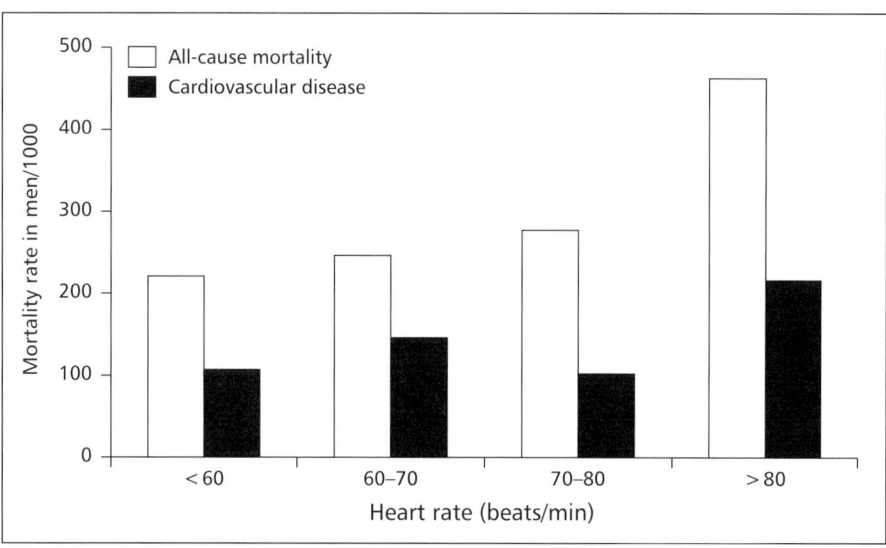

Figure 5 Mortality rate/1000 men aged 60–80 years according to initial heart rate (1982 to 1994)

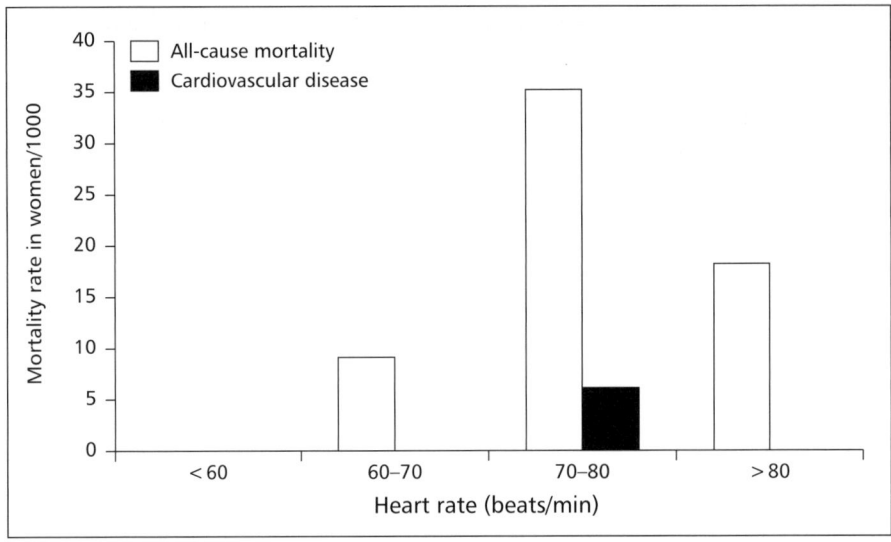

Figure 6 Mortality rate/1000 women aged 40–60 years according to initial heart rate (1982 to 1994)

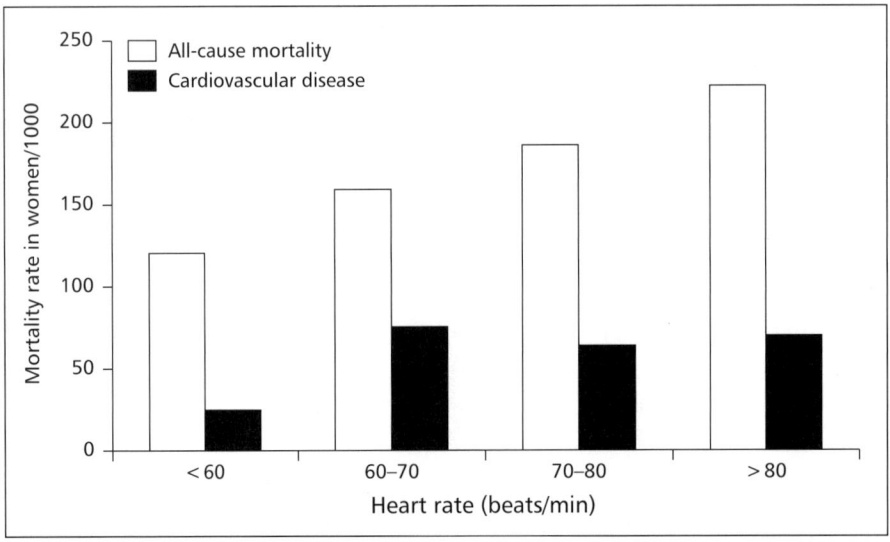

Figure 7 Mortality rate/1000 women aged 60–80 years according to initial heart rate (1982 to 1994)

PHARMACOLOGICAL REDUCTION OF HEART RATE

In view of the persistence of anginal attacks despite optimal treatment,[33] additional therapeutic approaches are required. In this connection, treatment (such as β-blockers) that decreases heart rate has been reported to reduce mortality and improve the outcome of ischemic heart disease.[51] It appears that there is often an almost linear relationship between reduction in mortality and reduction in heart rate during treatment with β-blockers, while drugs that do not reduce heart rate after MI do not improve survival. It was, therefore, proposed that decrease in heart rate should be an objective of the treatment of ischemic cardiovascular disease.[36]

The mechanisms by which heart rate reduction provides protection against myocardial ischemia are considered to reflect, in part, reduced myocardial oxygen requirement and increased diastolic perfusion time.[56] Since β-blockers have negative inotropic properties and may produce coronary arterial vasoconstriction, selective bradycardic drugs have been used to reduce heart rate without exerting these types of adverse actions.

The agents that have been used to produce bradycardia inhibit the hyperpolarization-activated I_f channel of the pacemaker cells of the sinoatrial node.[33] The drugs, such as ivabradine, increase the duration of spontaneous depolarization and produce a selective reduction in heart rate,[56] resulting in dose-dependent reduction in heart rate at rest and during exercise.[57] In this context, ivabradine has been reported to reduce heart rate exclusively and improve exercise capacity in patients with stable angina.[58,59]

SUMMARY

In summary, the prevalence of stable angina increases with age, loss of cardioprotective estrogen effects, and presence of risk factors such as hypertension, high cholesterol levels, physical inactivity and obesity. Although mortality from cardiovascular disease has decreased during the past few decades, further reduction is needed. The recognition of resting heart rate as an independent risk factor, and the development of treatments specifically designed to lower resting heart rate, provide a signpost for future advances. Successful management of chronic stable angina is important not only because of the high prevalence of the disease, of its social costs and its impact on individual quality of life, but also because of the considerable associated morbidity and mortality in the elderly population.

REFERENCES

1.   The American College of Cardiology/American Heart Association Task Force on Practice Guidelines. ACC/AHA 2002 Guideline Update for the Management of Patients With Chronic Stable Angina. 2002. Accessed Oct 25th, 2004. http://www.acc.org/clinical/guidelines/stable/update_index.htm

2.   Management of stable angina pectoris. Recommendations of the Task Force of the European Society of Cardiology, *Eur Heart J*. 1997;18:394–413.

3.   Tanne D, Shotan A, Goldbourt U et al. Severity of angina pectoris and risk of ischemic stroke. *Stroke*. 2002;33:245–250

4.   Kannel WB, Wolf PA, Verter J. Manifestations of coronary disease predisposing to stroke. The Framingham study. *JAMA*. 1983;250:2942–2946

5.   Elveback LR, Connolly DC, Melton LJ, 3rd. Coronary heart disease in residents of Rochester, Minnesota. VII. Incidence, 1950 through 1982. *Mayo Clin Proc*. 1986;61:896–900

6.   Kannel WB, Feinleib M. Natural history of angina pectoris in the Framingham study. Prognosis and survival. *Am J Cardiol*. 1972;29:154–163

7.   The American Heart Association. Heart disease and stroke statistics update. Dallas: American Heart Association, 2004

8.   Gandhi MM, Lampe FC, Wood DA. Incidence, clinical characteristics, and short-term prognosis of angina pectoris. *Br Heart J*. 1995;73:193–198

9.   Fenton DE, Baumann BM. Acute Coronary Syndrome. 2004. Accessed October 27th, 2004. http://www.emedicine.com/emerg/byname/acute-coronary-syndrome.htm

10.   Nilsson S, Scheike M, Engblom D, et al. Chest pain and ischaemic heart disease in primary care. *Br J Gen Pract*. 2003;53:378–382

11.   Joseph AM, Fu SS. Smoking cessation for patients with cardiovascular disease: what is the best approach? *Am J Cardiovasc Drugs*. 2003;3:339–349

12.   Goldenberg I, Jonas M, Tenenbaum A et al. Current smoking, smoking cessation, and the risk of sudden cardiac death in patients with coronary artery disease. *Arch Intern Med*. 2003;163:2301–2305

13.   Higgins M, Kannel W, Garrison R et al. Hazards of obesity—the Framingham experience. *Acta Med Scand*. Suppl 1988;723:23–36

14.   Kannel WB, Wilson PW, Nam BH, D'Agostino RB. Risk stratification of obesity as a coronary risk factor. *Am J Cardiol*. 2002;90:697–701

15.   Tseng CH. Body composition as a risk factor for coronary artery disease in Chinese type 2 diabetic patients in Taiwan. *Circ J*. 2003;67:479–484

16. Welborn TA, Dhaliwal SS, Bennett SA. Waist–hip ratio is the dominant risk factor predicting cardiovascular death in Australia. *Med J Aust*. 2003;179:580–585

17. Zhu S, St-Onge MP, Heshka S, Heymsfield SB. Lifestyle behaviors associated with lower risk of having the metabolic syndrome. *Metabolism*. 2004;53:1503–1511

18. Li JJ, Fang CH. C-reactive protein is not only an inflammatory marker but also a direct cause of cardiovascular diseases. *Med Hypotheses*. 2004;62:499–506

19. Hoshida S, Nishino M, Takeda T et al. A persistent increase in C-reactive protein is a risk factor for restenosis in patients with stable angina who are not receiving statins. *Atherosclerosis*. 2004;173:285–290

20. Arroyo-Espliguero R, Avanzas P, Cosin-Sales J et al. C-reactive protein elevation and disease activity in patients with coronary artery disease. *Eur Heart J*. 2004;25:401–408

21. Jukema JW, Bruschke AV, van Boven AJ et al. Effects of lipid lowering by pravastatin on progression and regression of coronary artery disease in symptomatic men with normal to moderately elevated serum cholesterol levels. The Regression Growth Evaluation Statin Study (REGRESS). *Circulation*. 1995;91:2528–2540

22. MacMahon S, Sharpe N, Gamble G et al. Effects of lowering average of below-average cholesterol levels on the progression of carotid atherosclerosis: results of the LIPID Atherosclerosis Substudy. LIPID Trial Research Group. *Circulation*. 1998;97:1784–1790

23. MRC/BHF Heart Protection Study of cholesterol lowering with simvastatin in 20,536 high-risk individuals: a randomised placebo-controlled trial. *Lancet*. 2002;360:7–22

24. Pocock SJ, Shaper AG, Phillips AN. Concentrations of high density lipoprotein cholesterol, triglycerides, and total cholesterol in ischaemic heart disease. *Br Med J*. 1989;298:998–1002

25. Grundy SM, Cleeman JI, Merz CN et al. Implications of recent clinical trials for the National Cholesterol Education Program Adult Treatment Panel III guidelines. *Arterioscler Thromb Vasc Biol*. 2004;24:e149–e161

26. Julien J. Cardiac complications in non-insulin-dependent diabetes mellitus. *J Diabetes Complications*. 1997;11:123–130

27. Wannamethee SG, Shaper AG, Lennon L. Cardiovascular disease incidence and mortality in older men with diabetes and in men with coronary heart disease. *Heart*. 2004;90:1398–1403

28. Capewell S, Beaglehole R, Seddon M, McMurray J. Explanation for the decline in coronary heart disease mortality rates in Auckland, New Zealand, between 1982 and 1993. *Circulation*. 2000;102:1511–1516

29. Glader EL, Stegmayr B. Declining prevalence of angina pectoris in middle-aged men and women. A population-based study within the Northern Sweden MONICA Project. Multinational Monitoring of Trends and Cardiovascular Disease. *J Intern Med*. 1999;246:285–291

30. D'Agostino RB, Kannel WB, Belanger AJ, Sytkowski PA. Trends in CHD and risk factors at age 55–64 in the Framingham Study. *Int J Epidemiol*. 1989;18:S67–S72

31. Australian Bureau of Statistics. Year Book Australia. Cardiovascular disease: 30th century trends. http: //www.abs.au 2003

32. Greenland P, Daviglus ML, Dyer AR et al. Resting heart rate is a risk factor for cardiovascular and noncardiovascular mortality: the Chicago Heart Association Detection Project in Industry. *Am J Epidemiol*. 1999;149:853–862

33. Borer JS. Drug insight: I_f inhibitors as specific heart-rate-reducing agents. *Cardiovasc Med*. 2004;1:103–109

34. Okamura T, Hayakawa T, Kadowaki T et al. (NIPPONDATA80 Research Group.) Resting heart rate and cause-specific death in a 16.5-year cohort study of the Japanese general population. *Am Heart J*. 2004;147:1024–1032

35. Hozawa A, Ohkubo T, Kikuya M et al. Prognostic value of home heart rate for cardiovascular mortality in the general population: the Ohasama study. *Am J Hypertens*. 2004;17:1005–1010

36. Laperche T, Logeart D, Cohen-Solal A, Gourgon R. Potential interests of heart rate lowering drugs. *Heart*. 1999;81:336–341

37. Levine HJ. Rest heart rate and life expectancy. *J Am Coll Cardiol*. 1997;30: 1104–1106

38. Kaplan JR, Manuck SB, Clarkson TB. The influence of heart rate on coronary artery atherosclerosis. *J Cardiovasc Pharmacol*. 1987;10 Suppl 2:S100–S102; discussion S3

39. Beere PA, Glagov S, Zarins CK. Retarding effect of lowered heart rate on coronary atherosclerosis. *Science*. 1984;226:180–182

40. Benetos A, Rudnichi A, Thomas F et al. Influence of heart rate on mortality in a French population: role of age, gender, and blood pressure. *Hypertension*. 1999;33:44–52

41. Mensink GB, Hoffmeister H. The relationship between resting heart rate and all-cause, cardiovascular and cancer mortality. *Eur Heart J*. 1997;18:1404–1410

42. Kannel WB, Kannel C, Paffenbarger RS, Jr., Cupples LA. Heart rate and cardiovascular mortality: the Framingham Study. *Am Heart J*. 1987;113:1489–1494

43. Palatini P. Heart rate as a cardiovascular risk factor: do women differ from men? *Ann Med*. 2001;33:213–221

44. Palatini P, Casiglia E, Julius S, Pessina AC. High heart rate: a risk factor for cardiovascular death in elderly men. *Arch Intern Med*. 1999;159:585–592

45. Okamura T, Hayakawa T, Kadowaki T, et al. Prognostic value of home heart rate for cardiovascular mortality in the general population. The Ohasama study. *Am J Hypertens*. 2004;17:1005–1010

46. Hjalmarson A, Gilpin EA, Kjekshus J et al. Influence of heart rate on mortality after acute myocardial infarction. *Am J Cardiol*. 1990;65:547–553

47. Kristal-Boneh E, Silber H, Harari G, Froom P. The association of resting heart rate with cardiovascular, cancer and all-cause mortality. Eight year follow-up of 3527 male Israeli employees (the CORDIS Study). *Eur Heart J*. 2000;21:116–124

48. Kjekshus JK. Importance of heart rate in determining beta-blocker efficacy in acute and long-term acute myocardial infarction intervention trials. *Am J Cardiol*. 1986;57:43F–49F

49. Perski A, Hamsten A, Lindvall K, Theorell T. Heart rate correlates with severity of coronary atherosclerosis in young postinfarction patients. *Am Heart J*. 1988;116:1369–1373

50. Shaper AG, Wannamethee G, Macfarlane PW, Walker M. Heart rate, ischaemic heart disease, and sudden cardiac death in middle-aged British men. *Br Heart J*. 1993;70:49–55

51. Hjalmarson A. Significance of reduction in heart rate in cardiovascular disease. *Clin Cardiol*. 1998;21:113–117

52. Wannamethee G, Shaper AG. The association between heart rate and blood pressure, blood lipids and other cardiovascular risk factors. *J Cardiovasc Risk*. 1994;1:223–230

53. Morcet JF, Safar M, Thomas F et al. Associations between heart rate and other risk factors in a large French population. *J Hypertens*. 1999;17:1671–1676

54. Bonaa KH, Arnesen E. Association between heart rate and atherogenic blood lipid fractions in a population. The Tromso Study. *Circulation*. 1992;86:394–405

55. Perski A, Olsson G, Landou C et al. Minimum heart rate and coronary atherosclerosis: independent relations to global severity and rate of progression of angiographic lesions in men with myocardial infarction at a young age. *Am Heart J*. 1992;123:609–616

56. Monnet X, Ghaleh B, Colin P et al. Effects of heart rate reduction with ivabradine on exercise-induced myocardial ischemia and stunning. *J Pharmacol Exp Ther*. 2001;299:1133–1139

57. Colin P, Ghaleh B, Hittinger L et al. Differential effects of heart rate reduction and beta-blockade of left ventricular relaxation during exercise. *Am J Physiol Heart Circ Physiol*. 2002;282:H672–H679

58. DiFrancesco D, Camm JA. Heart rate lowering by specific and selective I(f) current inhibition with ivabradine: a new therapeutic perspective in cardiovascular disease. *Drugs*. 2004;64:1757–1765

59. Borer JS, Fox K. Jaillon P, et al. Antianginal and antiischemic effects of ivabradine and I_f inhibitor, in stable angina. A randomized, double-blind multicentered, placebo-controlled trial. *Circulation*. 2003;107:817–823

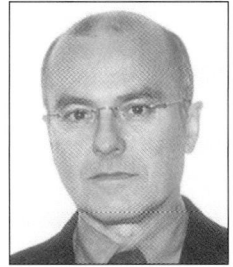

José López-Sendón

2 Goals for optimal treatment of patients with stable angina, and limits of current treatments

*José López-Sendón, †Caroline A Daly,
‡Esteban López de Sá

*Cardiology Department
Hospital Universitario La Paz
Pº de la Castellana 261
28046 Madrid, Spain
Tel: +34 91 586 8295
Fax: +34 91 586 8292
Email: jlsendon@terra.es

†Cardiology Department
Royal Brompton Hospital
Sydney Street, London, SW3 9NP, UK

‡Coronary Care Unit
Hospital Universitario Gregorio Marañón
Doctor Esquerdo 46
28007 Madrid, Spain

INTRODUCTION

Stable angina pectoris is a clinical syndrome characterized by chest pain or discomfort that is secondary to myocardial ischemia and is without the clinical features associated with instability.[1-3] Usually, stable angina is secondary to significant stenosis of the coronary arteries, impairing coronary flow and myocardial perfusion, and angina is triggered by factors that increase myocardial oxygen consumption, such as exercise, tachycardia or hypertension; however, any factor associated with an imbalance between myocardial oxygen supply and consumption can induce angina, even in the absence of significant coronary artery lesions (e.g. anemia, aortic stenosis, ventricular hypertrophy, arrhythmias) (*Figure 1*). A distinctive feature of this clinical syndrome is stability. Recent-onset symptoms (usually less than a month), prolonged (more than 20 minutes) or progressive (increasing severity by at least one functional class and at least to functional class III angina), recent myocardial infarction and resting angina are the typical features associated with instability,[4] which exclude the diagnosis of *stable* angina and constitute a medical emergency. In other words, *stable* angina is angina *without* instability criteria. Silent ischemia[5] and stable chronic ischemic heart disease[1,2] are related to stable angina, the distinctive feature of angina being the presence of chest pain or discomfort. Chronic stable angina pectoris is a common and disabling disorder. Its prevalence varies, reaching 11–20% in the 65–74 year age group for men, this increases rapidly with age and is related to prognosis.[1,3]

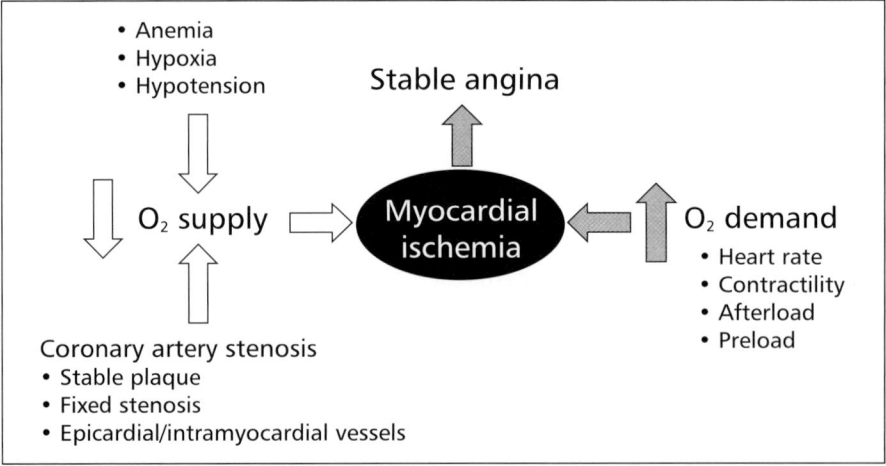

Figure 1 Myocardial ischemia is the consequence of an imbalance between myocardial oxygen supply and consumption. Stable angina is secondary to ischemia triggered by factors that increase myocardial oxygen consumption in the presence of fixed, stable coronary stenosis

ASSESSMENT OF PATIENTS WITH STABLE ANGINA

Treatment of patients with stable angina should be directed not only at controlling symptoms or identifying and treating coronary stenosis, but a complete evaluation of the patient is also mandatory, and should always include a correct diagnosis, investigation of possible associated conditions, gradation of the severity of ischemia, characterization of the risk profile and identification of possible contraindications for medical or invasive treatment (Table 1).[1–3]

Table 1 Evaluation of patients with stable angina

Correct diagnosis of angina
    Identify ischemia
    Exclude other causes of angina

Characterization of risk profile
    Severity of ischemia
    Ventricular function
    Other (age, diabetes)

Identification of aggravating/precipitating causes
    Hypertension
    Arrhythmias (atrial fibrillation, tachycardia)
    Anemia

Identify possible contraindications for medical/revascularization treatment
    Bradycardia
    Hypotension
    Renal failure

Diagnosis of angina is based on the clinical symptoms, but other causes of chest pain must be ruled out and some evidence of ischemia must be demonstrated, especially in patients without typical symptoms and in the absence of a previous history of ischemic heart disease. A resting 12-lead electrocardiogram (ECG) may be normal in a significant proportion of cases, but may also reveal dynamic ST-segment changes in the presence of ischemia, particularly if there is an opportunity to obtain tracings with and without the presence of pain.[6] An exercise stress test, with or without imaging techniques, is certainly more sensitive and specific for the diagnosis of ischemia, and is recommended in the initial evaluation of all patients with suspected stable angina.[7,8] Coronary angiography for diagnostic purposes should be reserved for high-risk patients and those without appropriate control of angina symptoms.[1,3] Other causes of angina, such as aortic stenosis and hypertrophic cardiomyopathy, must be routinely excluded, as well as conditions that may precipitate or aggravate ischemia, including anemia, hypertension and arrhythmias, especially atrial fibrillation and tachycardia.[1,3]

The prognosis of patients with stable angina is variable, and risk stratification facilitates the selection of treatment options, in particular the need for coronary artery angiography and revascularization.[1,3] The strongest predictor for outcome is ventricular function (left ventricular ejection fraction).[9] However, other important information for appropriate risk stratification is derived from the clinical profile of the patient, including age, female gender, previous history of any cardiovascular disease, co-morbidity conditions, the severity of angina,[10] the presence and severity of classical cardiovascular risk factors (smoking, diabetes, hypertension and hyperlipidemia)[11,12] and ECG abnormalities (previous myocardial infarction, ST-segment depression) in the resting ECG.[13] Response to stress testing has been given special attention, and some risk scores that consider the presence and severity of stress-induced ischemia have been developed, the most popular being that proposed by Duke University.[14] Finally, the extent and severity of coronary artery disease are important independent indicators of long-term outcome; left main stem, three-vessel disease, and proximal, left-anterior, descending severe stenosis and its combinations have consistently been identified as the most important coronary lesions associated with the worst outcome.[15] Although there is no well-defined and validated risk score, patients with stable angina can be categorized into three broad groups, with a low, intermediate or high risk of suffering cardiovascular events during long-term evolution.

GOALS OF TREATMENT

After the diagnosis and characterization of stable angina have been completed, the three main goals of treatment include: relief of pain during the ischemic episodes; control of symptoms; and improvement in outcome, the latter being closely related to secondary prevention of ischemic heart disease (Table 2).

Table 2 Goals of treatment in patients with stable angina

Immediate pain relief

Control of angina

    Reduce/control ischemic episodes

    Improve functional capacity

Secondary prevention

    Reduce progression of cardiovascular disease

    Reduce morbidity

    Prolong survival

Relief of pain

Immediate relief of pain during ischemic episodes is achieved, in most cases, by simply discontinuing the activity (usually exercise) that has induced the episode. If this fails, sublingual administration of nitrates is very effective; if pain still persists, or changes pattern, the patient must be instructed to seek urgent medical advice.

Control of angina

Control of angina implies the abolishment or reduction in the number of ischemic episodes, improving functional capacity and allowing a normal life. The first step towards this goal is the control of aggravating or precipitating factors and associated conditions related to the ischemic episodes; these include hypertension or hypotension, anemia, arrhythmias and factors associated with an increase in myocardial oxygen consumption.

Medical treatment

Effective medical treatments for reducing ischemia and improving functional capacity include β-blockers, calcium channel blockers, nitrates, potassium channel openers and late sodium current inhibitors. Surprisingly, there is relatively little information about the efficacy of anti-anginal drugs, compared with the extensive experience in clinical trials of other ischemic syndromes, including myocardial infarction and unstable angina. For this reason, the selection of drugs is based on general information obtained across the full spectrum of cardiovascular diseases (Table 3).

Table 3 Treatment of patients with stable angina

Immediate pain relief
Immediate rest and sublingual nitrates. Instruct the patient
Seek urgent medical advice if pain not relieved in minutes or changes pattern

Control of angina
Control precipitation/aggravating factors and associated conditions
β-blockers preferred as first-line treatment, especially if previous myocardial
    infarction or impaired ventricular function
Change to other anti-ischemic drug if β-blockers contraindicated or not
    tolerated (non-dihydropyridine Ca channel blocker as preferred choice)
Add other anti-ischemic drug if angina/ischemia not well controlled
Consider revascularization if angina not well controlled and in high-risk patients

Secondary prevention
Lifestyle changes
    avoid toxic habits; cease smoking
    healthy diet (Mediterranean)
    regular exercise

Control/treatment of major risk factors
    Hypertension
    Diabetes
    Dyslipidemia. Goal: low-density lipoprotein < 100 (statins first choice)

Aspirin in all; clopidogrel in patients intolerant to aspirin
Statins in most patients with confirmed cardiovascular disease
Angiotensin-converting enzyme inhibitors if proven vascular disease, and
    intermediate- or high-risk for cardiovascular events

β-blockers are the preferred choice as first-line treatment in the absence of contraindications, especially in patients with previous myocardial infarction or impaired ventricular function.[1–3,16] β-blockers reduce the episodes of angina, improve functional capacity and, in patients with previous myocardial infarction or heart failure, reduce long-term mortality,[16] a clinical benefit not observed with any of the other drugs recommended for the treatment of stable angina. If a β-blocker is contraindicated or not well tolerated, non-dihydropyridine calcium channel blockers that also reduce heart rate could be the best choice.[17] If the angina is not well controlled despite the correct use of β-blockers, the recommendation is to add another anti-ischemic drug, either a dihydropyridine calcium channel blocker[18] or a long-acting nitrate,[19] a potassium channel opener (nicorandil)[20] or a metabolic agent such as trimetazidine, the first 3-KAT inhibitor, which provides benefits in patients with stable angina.[21] Forthcoming products include the late sodium current inhibitor ranolazine;[22] furthermore, the selective and specific I_f current inhibitor ivabradine, has proven to be an efficient anti-ischemic and anti-anginal agent, while exclusively reducing heart rate.[23] All these agents have demonstrated some benefit in stable angina, mainly a reduction in ischemic episodes and an improvement in exercise capacity; however, no further clinical benefits have been observed in clinical trials, except with the use of nicorandil. Two recent large clinical trials in patients with stable angina deserve some comment. In the IONA trial, with nicorandil added to standard therapy, there was a reduction in the combined clinical endpoint of death by infarction or hospitalization for heart failure.[20] In the ACTION trial, long-acting nifedipine was compared with placebo in over 7000 patients; no difference in the combined endpoint for clinical efficacy was found between the active drug and placebo after 5-years' follow-up.[24]

Coronary artery revascularization

Coronary artery revascularization is indicated when control of angina is insufficient, as well as in high-risk patients.[1,3] The prognostic benefit of surgical revascularization, compared with medical therapy, has not been demonstrated in low-risk patients. However, in high-risk patients (e.g. those with severe ischemia and impaired left ventricular function) surgery may improve prognosis.[25] In addition, the presence of specific coronary artery anatomy (significant stenosis of the main stem and two- or three-vessel disease with proximal stenosis involving the left-anterior descending coronary artery) has been demonstrated to be associated with a better prognosis with surgery than with medical treatment.[25] Percutaneous coronary intervention rivals surgical revascularization procedures,[26] but again the benefit, compared with medical treatment, has not been demonstrated in low-risk patients with chronic stable coronary artery disease.

Secondary prevention

Secondary prevention has a very important role in patients with stable angina. Although there is no direct information in selected populations of patients with chronic stable angina, there is a strong recommendation for adherence to the secondary prevention guidelines.[1–3] Complete cessation of smoking,[27] regular exercise,[28] a healthy diet of the Mediterranean type,[29] as well as the treatment and control of major risk factors including hypertension[30] and dyslipidemias,[31] have been clearly associated with a reduction in cardiovascular complications and an improvement in survival.

For the same reasons, the routine, long-term use of aspirin[32] and statins[31,33] is recommended in all patients, and angiotensin-converting enzyme inhibitors in all but the low-risk group of patients with chronic ischemic heart disease and stable angina.[34,35]

LIMITATIONS OF CURRENT TREATMENTS

There is a clear need for further clinical research in patients with stable angina (Table 4). The current data available are insufficient to provide evidence of a benefit with most of the drugs currently in use. Most of the information available focuses on exercise capacity and not on clinical outcome. The majority of studies were conducted years ago, when coronary angiography and revascularization were not used as frequently as they are today, and secondary prevention strategies were not so strongly recommended. In a large number of patients, single anti-anginal drug therapy is clearly insufficient to control ischemia, and there is very limited information about drug combinations when monotherapy has failed.

Table 4 Limitations of current treatments

Lack of convincing evidence for outcome improvement

Benefit focused mainly on functional capacity

Most studies conducted many years ago

Insufficient control of ischemia

Scarce information with combinations of anti-anginal drugs

Frequent contraindications or intolerance to therapeutic doses

Frequent secondary effects

A significant number of patients present contraindications for the use of β-blockers, nitrates or calcium channel blockers, or simply do not tolerate the appropriate doses. Finally, some of the anti-anginal drugs currently used in large populations present severe limitations for long-term use; pharmacological tolerance (lack of effect) to transdermal nitrates is very common within days of use, and the nitrate night-free period recommended by some may be associated with a rebound phenomenon and an increase in ischemic episodes.[19] Furthermore, calcium channel blockers may precipitate heart failure.[36]

Continuing developments in revascularization procedures, as well as significant progress in medical treatment and secondary prevention, and active research into drugs with new mechanisms of action, will generate a need for large randomized trials comparing different treatment strategies in selected groups of patients and the relevant clinical outcomes, not only in terms of ischemia or functional capacity – this should be the aim of new treatment strategies.

REFERENCES

1. Fox K, for the members of the Task Force on the Management of Stable Angina Pectoris of the European Society of Cardiology. Guidelines on the management of stable angina pectoris. *Eur Heart J.* 2005; in press.

2. De Backer G, Ambrosioni E, Borch-Johnsen K, et al. European guidelines on cardiovascular disease prevention in clinical practice: third joint task force of European and other societies on cardiovascular disease prevention in clinical practice (constituted by representatives of eight societies and by invited experts). *Eur J Cardiovasc Prev Rehabil.* 2003;10:S1–S10.

3. Gibbons RJ, for the ACC/AHA/ACP-ASIM Task Force on Stable Angina Guidelines. ACC/AHA/ACP-ASIM guidelines for the management of patients with chronic stable angina: a report of the American College of Cardiology/American Heart Association Task Force on Practice Guidelines (Committee on Management of Patients With Chronic Stable Angina). *J Am Coll Cardiol.* 1999;33:2092–2197.

4. Braunwald E. Unstable angina. A classification. *Circulation.* 1989;80:410–414.

5. Cohn PF, Fox KM, Daly C. Silent myocardial ischemia. *Circulation.* 2003;108:1263–1277.

6. Kleber AG. ST-segment elevation in the electrocardiogram: a sign of myocardial ischemia. *Cardiovasc Res.* 2000;45:111–118.

7. Lee TH, Boucher CA. Clinical practice. Noninvasive tests in patients with stable coronary artery disease. *N Engl J Med.* 2001;344:1840–1845.

8. Gibbons RJ, Balady GJ, Bricker JT, et al. ACC/AHA 2002 guideline update for exercise testing: summary article. A report of the American College of Cardiology/American Heart Association Task Force on Practice Guidelines (Committee to Update the 1997 Exercise Testing Guidelines). *J Am Coll Cardiol.* 2002;40:1531–1540.

34. Yusuf S, Sleight P, Pogue J, et al. Effects of an angiotensin-converting-enzyme inhibitor, ramipril, on cardiovascular events in high-risk patients. The Heart Outcomes Prevention Evaluation Study Investigators. *N Engl J Med*. 2000; 342:145–153.

35. Fox KM. Efficacy of perindopril in reduction of cardiovascular events among patients with stable coronary artery disease: randomised, double-blind, placebo-controlled, multicentre trial (the EUROPA study). *Lancet*. 2003;362:782–788.

36. Turnbull F. Effects of different blood-pressure-lowering regimens on major cardiovascular events: results of prospectively-designed overviews of randomised trials. *Lancet*. 2003;362:1527–1535.

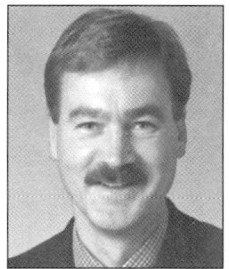

Gerd Heusch

3 The pathophysiological role of heart rate in acute myocardial ischemia and the benefits of heart rate reduction

Gerd Heusch, Rainer Schulz

Institut für Pathophysiologie
Universitätsklinikum Essen
Hufelandstr. 55
45122 Essen, Germany
Tel: +49 (201) 723 4480
Fax: +49 (201) 723 4481
E-mail: gerd.heusch@uni-essen.de

INTRODUCTION

It appears to be common wisdom that myocardial ischemia is characterized by an imbalance between supply and demand,[1] and that increased heart rate contributes to such an imbalance by both decreasing supply and increasing demand.

This view, however, is too simplistic, if not incorrect, largely because it does not adequately consider the regional nature of myocardial ischemia[2] in most clinical scenarios, with the exception of cardioplegic arrest where heart rate is of no importance. This review will characterize, in detail, both supply and demand in regional myocardial ischemia, and analyze the impact of heart rate thereon. The benefits resulting from pharmacological heart rate reduction will also be presented, and the potential advantages of agents that exclusively reduce heart rate will be highlighted.

METHODS FOR QUANTITATIVE ANALYSIS OF REGIONAL MYOCARDIAL BLOOD FLOW AND CONTRACTILE FUNCTION

Myocardial blood flow (perfusion)

The gold standard for the measurement of regional myocardial blood flow is the microspheres method.[3] This technique has a spatial resolution as low as < 100 mg of myocardial tissue, depending on the number of injected microspheres.[4,5] At this resolution, myocardial blood flow displays considerable heterogeneity, even during normoperfusion, with some areas having less than 20% of mean blood flow and others having more than 200%.[4,6,7] This spatial heterogeneity of myocardial blood flow is associated with a similar heterogeneity in oxidative metabolism[8–10] and protein expression.[11] Whether or not contractile function is similarly heterogeneous at such a microregional level is unclear at present (see below).[12] The major limitation of the microspheres technique is the limited number of radioactive or color tracers that can be used,[3,13] such that only a few sequential measurements can be made, and a continuous recording of regional blood flow is impossible.

The only currently available clinical method to measure regional myocardial blood flow quantitatively is positron emission tomography (PET).[14–16] However, PET has serious limitations, in addition to the expensive technical requirements and radiation safety concerns, that prevent its widespread and frequent use. PET flow measurements lack sufficient spatial (particularly transmural) resolution, and the lack of respiration- and/or cardiac motion-gated measurements exacerbates this problem, such that the spatial resolution is approximately 1 to 2 orders of magnitude less than that of the microspheres technique (i.e. 1 to 10 g, rather than 100 mg of myocardium). In addition, the very few normal blood flow values that have been reported from healthy volunteers vary widely (from $0.68 \pm 0.16 \, \text{ml} \, \text{g}^{-1} \, \text{min}^{-1}$ to $1.02 \pm 0.25 \, \text{ml} \, \text{g}^{-1} \, \text{min}^{-1}$ [mean $\pm$ SD]).[17,18] Consequently, in an individual patient, a major reduction in resting blood flow may go undetected, while only a modest reduction in transmural blood flow detected by PET in regions with contractile dysfunction may well translate to a much more severe reduction in subendocardial blood flow, which is the primary determinant of transmural wall function.[19] A further limitation is that PET, like the microspheres technique, does not permit continuous monitoring of myocardial blood flow, so most studies are only able to report data for a single timepoint only.

Myocardial contractile function (contraction)

The gold standard for the measurement of regional contractile function is sonomicrometry either of segment shortening or wall thickening.[20–22] A major advantage of sonomicrometry, in contrast to the flow measurement techniques described above, is that it allows continuous monitoring of contractile function. However, its spatial resolution is less than that of the microspheres technique by approximately an order of magnitude, although it can quantify differences between base and apex,[23,24] and particularly subendocardial and subepicardial contractile function.[19,25–27] In addition, sonomicrometry only measures wall excursion, not wall stress.[28] Severely hypokinetic and akinetic myocardium may develop substantial wall stress, such that the extent of contractile function and its associated metabolic cost are largely underestimated by sonomicrometric measurements of wall excursion only.[29–31] This consideration must be borne in mind, particularly when equating perfusion–contraction matching with energetic supply–demand.

Clinical methods to measure regional contractile function include echocardiography, contrast ventriculography, radionuclide ventriculography and magnetic resonance tomography. As with sonomicrometry, these clinical techniques also neglect wall stress. For obvious reasons, continuous measurements of regional contractile function, although technically possible with echocardiography, are unfeasible. Considering the technical limitations outlined above, it is immediately apparent that no combination of techniques to measure regional myocardial blood flow and function has sufficient spatial and temporal resolution to truly quantify their relationship over time during the development of myocardial ischemia.

QUANTITATIVE RELATIONSHIP BETWEEN PERFUSION AND CONTRACTION IN NORMAL AND ISCHEMIC MYOCARDIUM

Normoperfusion

In the normal heart, increases in contractile function are associated with increased metabolism, and the enhanced metabolic demands are met by increased oxygen extraction and, to a larger extent, by increased myocardial blood flow.[32,33] The mechanisms and mediators of such metabolic coronary dilation are still unclear,[32] but clearly perfusion–contraction matching is involved,[34] where alterations in contractile function are the cause of alterations in blood flow. Whether or not perfusion–contraction matching is also of relevance at the microregional level – i.e., whether or not the substantial spatial heterogeneity of myocardial blood flow is associated with a similar spatial heterogeneity of contractile function – is currently unclear, due to the insufficient spatial resolution of current techniques to measure contractile function.

A reverse causal relationship, whereby increases in myocardial blood flow cause increases in contractile function, does not exist in the normal beating heart.[35]

Acute ischemia

Following acute coronary artery inflow reduction, contractile function in the ischemic region is rapidly decreased.[36] As soon as a steady state has developed (after 2–3 min), enabling measurement of regional myocardial blood flow with the microspheres technique, a consistent relationship between the reduced regional contractile function is apparent. Vatner[37] was the first to demonstrate an exponential relationship between subendocardial blood flow and subendocardial segment shortening. Subsequently, Weintraub *et al.*[38] characterized the relationship between subendocardial blood flow and subendocardial segment shortening as sigmoidal, and Gallagher *et al.* found that the relationship between systolic wall thickening and subendocardial or transmural blood flow was more or less linear (*Figure 1*).[39,40] Whereas the shape of this flow–function relationship has been a matter of some controversy in the past, it is now considered that the consistent, close perfusion–contraction matching is more important than the apparent subtle differences in the shape of such a relationship, which may be attributable to differences in experimental conditions, segment shortening vs. wall thickening, data presentation and statistical phenomena.

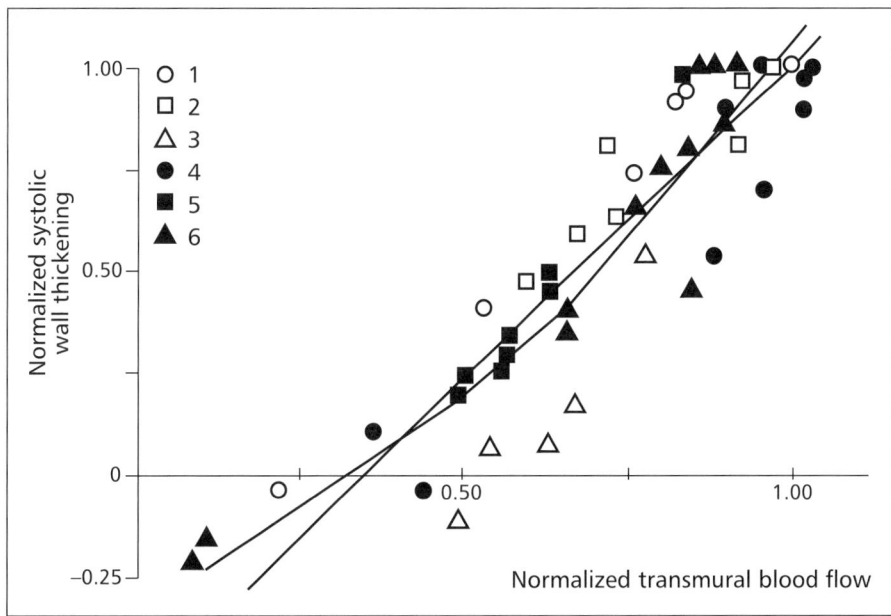

Figure 1 Linear relationship between normalized (as a fraction of baseline) regional myocardial systolic wall thickening and normalized (as a fraction of that in remote control myocardium) myocardial blood flow, i.e. perfusion–contraction matching. From Gallagher et al.[40]

The relationship between ischemic regional myocardial blood flow and contractile function varies with the hemodynamic situation. There is greater blood flow for a given level of function during exercise than when at rest.[39] However, when myocardial blood flow is normalized for heart rate (expressed as blood flow per beat rather than per minute, and thus related to the same temporal reference as contractile function – i.e. one arbitrary, average cardiac cycle), the relationships at rest and during exercise,[39] and those at different heart rates,[41,42] are superimposable. When equating such perfusion–contraction matching in acutely ischemic myocardium with an energetic supply–demand balance, several limitations must be considered. On the supply side, changes in myocardial oxygen extraction and anaerobic glycolytic metabolism may also contribute to supply, in addition to blood flow. On the demand side, regional wall excursion may underestimate the regional metabolic demand when the ischemic myocardium still develops wall tension, and indeed even dyskinetic myocardium has a surprisingly high oxygen consumption.[29–31,43]

The mechanisms and biochemical signals that underlie the rapid development of perfusion–contraction matching in acutely ischemic myocardium remain unclear. Endogenous nitric oxide (NO) is not the biochemical signal for perfusion–contraction matching, but sets the level for such matching; i.e., with inhibition of NO synthesis, regional myocardial function for any level of blood flow and oxygen consumption is reduced in anesthetized, open-chest[44] and sedated, chronically instrumented pigs[45] subjected to 90 min of acute ischemia.

DISTRIBUTION OF PERFUSION AND CONTRACTION BETWEEN ISCHEMIC AND NON-ISCHEMIC MYOCARDIUM

Perfusion

Whereas collaterals certainly have a cardioprotective function,[46,47] they can also be the underlying morphological substrate for aggravation of myocardial ischemia when steal phenomena occur. In the presence of a flow-limiting coronary stenosis, flow into the ischemic terminal vascular bed is the sum of coronary arterial inflow through the stenosis and collateral inflow from adjacent non-ischemic or less ischemic regions (*Figure 2*). Collateral inflow is dependent on the pressure gradient between the origin of collaterals in the intact donor vessels and their orifice into the ischemic recipient vessels. When the dilator reserve of the ischemic recipient vessels is fully exhausted, and flow is therefore pressure-dependent, any dilation of the non-ischemic, donor terminal vascular bed during enhanced metabolic demand,[48] or in response to dilator agents,[49–53] will decrease the driving pressure gradient across the collaterals and, in consequence, collateral flow. This phenomenon has been termed 'collateral steal'.[54] A similar situation is evident with respect to the transmural distribution of myocardial blood flow when the subendocardial autoregulatory reserve is exhausted but some subepicardial autoregulatory reserve persists.[55] The dilation of sub epicardial vessels during enhanced metabolic demand will then compromise subendocardial perfusion,[56] a phenomenon termed 'transmural steal'. This phenomenon can be considered as the major cause of the preferential subendocardial manifestation of myocardial ischemia and infarction. Finally, a steal situation also develops when a stenotic coronary artery perfuses parts of both left and right ventricles. During increased myocardial metabolic demand, a redistribution from the left to the right ventricular perfusion territory – i.e. a right-ventricular steal phenomenon – may occur.[57] The presence of a well-developed collateral circulation often maintains sufficient blood flow to the post-stenotic myocardium at rest, but steal phenomena contribute to the precipitation of myocardial ischemia during exercise.[58–60]

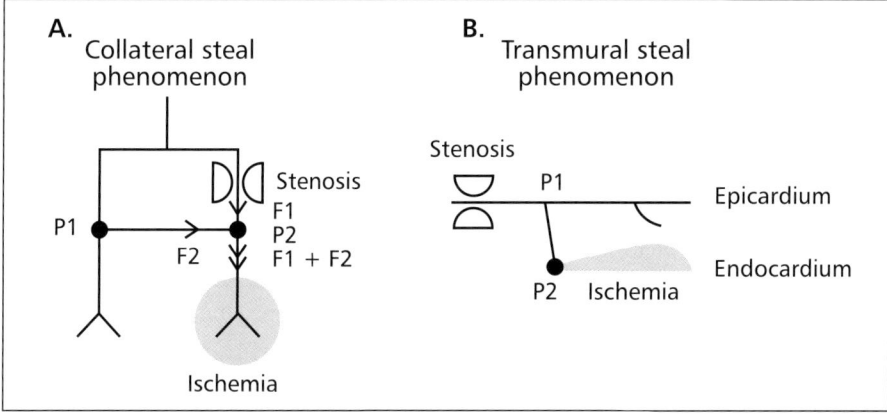

Figure 2 Collateral (A) and transmural (B) steal phenomena. P1 = pressure at the origin of collaterals, P2 = pressure at the orifice of collaterals into the ischemic terminal vascular bed, F1 = flow through the stenosis, F2 = collateral blood flow. Any dilation of the normal terminal vascular bed will decrease P1 and, consequently, the gradient P1–P2 and finally F2. From Baumgart et al.[61]

Contraction

Regional ischemic dysfunction has been characterized above, but regional myocardial ischemia also impacts on the non-ischemic myocardium. During acute coronary artery occlusion in anesthetized swine,[62] and in both anesthetized[63] and conscious dogs,[64,65] the ischemic region is surrounded by a narrow zone of normally perfused myocardium with depressed systolic wall thickening or segment shortening. This depressed contractile function in the immediate border zone surrounding the ischemic region is attributed to more or less well-defined mechanical 'tethering' between non-ischemic and ischemic myocardial fibers.[66] The mechanism of such tethering is probably related to the existence of high regional wall stresses present at the border between ischemic and dysfunctional vs. normal myocardium.[67] Such a dysfunctional border zone leads to overestimation of the ischemic region, from a diagnostic point of view.

A dysfunctional, non-ischemic border zone may not only extend laterally from an ischemic region during complete coronary occlusion, but also overlie the ischemic inner myocardial layers during non-transmural ischemia. The subepicardium becomes dysfunctional if ischemia is restricted to the subendocardium and subepicardial perfusion is normal,[25,68] and outer wall dysfunction is disproportional to the outer wall flow reduction during treadmill exercise in dogs with coronary stenosis.[69]

Whereas lateral and transmural tethering create a non-ischemic, dysfunctional border zone in the immediate vicinity of the ischemic region, more remote non-ischemic regions are characterized by enhanced contractile function.[70–73] Whether an increase in remote non-ischemic zone function can be considered as compensatory in that it acts to preserve global left ventricular (LV) function[70,73,74] is not completely clear, since a major part of non-ischemic zone hyperfunction occurs during isovolumic systole and does not contribute to ejection.[71] The increase in function in the remote non-ischemic zone is associated with a moderate, presumably metabolically mediated, increase in blood flow to this region.[70,75] However, the relationship of regional myocardial blood flow and function in remote, hyperfunctioning, non-ischemic myocardium has not yet been systematically analyzed.

EFFECTS OF HEART RATE ON PERFUSION AND CONTRACTION IN NORMAL AND ISCHEMIC MYOCARDIUM

An increase in heart rate increases the number of cardiac cycles per timeframe and, therefore, the energy/oxygen demand per timeframe (*Figure 3*). In addition, in some species, possibly including man, an increase in heart rate increases the myocardial inotropic state through a force–frequency effect.[76] With intact coronary circulation, metabolic vasodilation serves to increase coronary blood flow to match the increased oxygen demand, since myocardial oxygen extraction is near maximal at baseline and can only be increased by a small amount. Simultaneously with increasing oxygen demand, an increase in heart rate also shortens diastolic duration, and thus the time interval of the cardiac cycle where almost all of the coronary blood flow occurs.[77,78] In intact coronary circulation, metabolic vasodilation is sufficiently powerful to overcome the limitation of coronary blood flow by reduced diastolic duration, such that the increased oxygen demand is adequately matched; thus, increased heart rate is associated with proportionately increased myocardial oxygen consumption. However, in the presence of a severe coronary stenosis, when the autoregulatory capacity of the coronary circulation is exhausted to maintain a normal coronary blood flow at baseline, any further increase in heart rate (or, more precisely, any further reduction in diastolic perfusion time[79]) will compromise coronary blood flow such that it is actually reduced at higher heart rates.

In the case of regional myocardial ischemia, where a severely stenotic coronary artery is connected via collaterals with an intact or less severely affected coronary artery, a typical redistribution/steal scenario develops, as outlined above: metabolic vasodilation of the more or less intact coronary microcirculation decreases collateral perfusion pressure and, in consequence, collateral blood flow into the post-stenotic coronary microcirculation is reduced[48] and ischemia is precipitated. In addition to such steal phenomenon, the hemodynamic severity of a coronary stenosis is increased at a higher heart rate because of increased turbulence, and this effect serves to further compromise coronary inflow.[80,81]

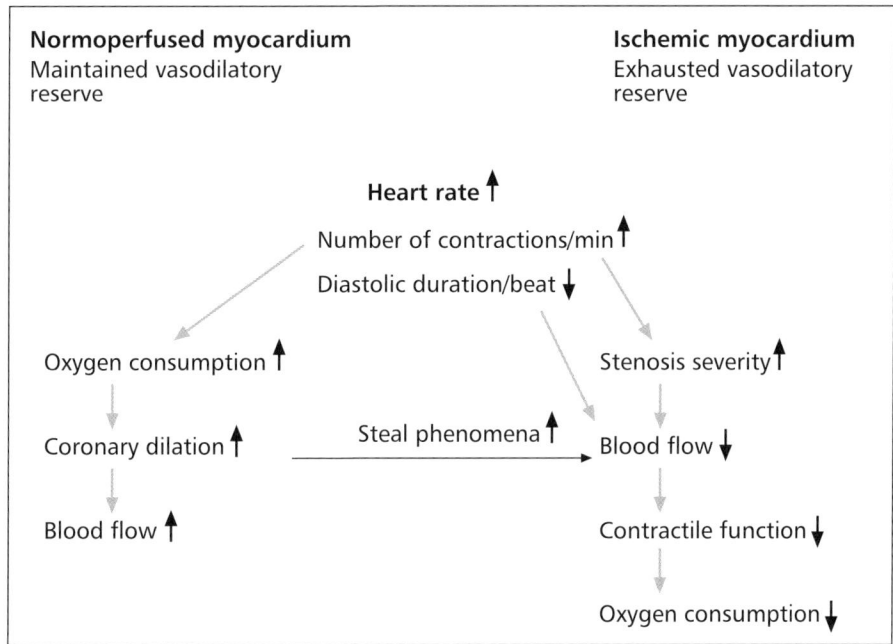

Figure 3 Schematic diagram depicting the effects of increased heart rate on myocardial flow, function and oxygen consumption

β-ADRENERGIC BLOCKADE IN REGIONAL MYOCARDIAL ISCHEMIA

Exercise and excitement are characterized by sympathetic activation, and β-adrenergic mechanisms contribute to myocardial ischemia through an unfavorable redistribution of coronary blood flow away from the ischemic subendocardium – i.e. through a collateral as well as a transmural steal mechanism (see above). β-blockade decreases heart rate at rest, and attenuates the exercise-induced increases in heart rate, LV dP/dt and function of the non-ischemic myocardium. In consequence, the increases in blood flow to the non-ischemic myocardium and the post-stenotic subepicardium are attenuated. However, subendocardial blood flow of the ischemic myocardium is increased, resulting in improved regional myocardial function.[82]

The hemodynamic severity of a dynamic coronary stenosis is reduced by β-blockade. The β-blockade-induced autoregulatory decrease in flow to non-ischemic regions results in an increase in post-stenotic coronary perfusion pressure. Increased perfusion pressure, in turn, reduces stenotic resistance, thus finally improving blood flow to ischemic regions.[83] The beneficial effects of β-blockade in exercise-induced myocardial ischemia are almost exclusively due to the attenuation of the increase in heart rate. When this reduction in heart rate is prevented by atrial pacing, ischemic regional myocardial blood flow and function are slightly reduced, compared with the untreated situation, possibly because of an unmasking of α-adrenergic constriction in the ischemic coronary microcirculation.[59] The disadvantage of β-blockade, in reducing the inotropic state, is well established; however, the importance of α-adrenergic coronary vasoconstriction in patients with stable angina, or in patients undergoing coronary interventions,[84–87] is currently largely neglected or underestimated.

CLINICAL EVIDENCE FOR BENEFIT FROM HEART RATE REDUCTION

A subanalysis of data from the Framingham study in 2037 men and 2493 women with a blood pressure > 140/90 mmHg demonstrated that there was a 20% increase in overall mortality and a 14% increase in cardiovascular mortality in both genders, after adjustment for age and blood pressure.[88] The British Regional Heart Study (BRHS) prospectively followed up 7335 men with ischemic heart disease, and revealed a strong association between resting heart rate and major ischemic cardiac events, including death and sudden cardiac death.[89] Similarly, a positive association between elevated heart rate and cardiovascular death was reported in the CASTEL study.[90] In patients with acute myocardial infarction, there was a positive association between heart rate at admission and total mortality. Total mortality rates were 15%, 41% and 48% for patients with admission heart rates of 50 to 60/min, > 90/min and >110/min, respectively.[91] Similar findings were reported from the GISSI-2 study for patients undergoing thrombolysis.[92]

The concept of heart rate reduction having a beneficial effect is also supported by three further studies that clearly documented reduced mortality in patients with heart failure when treated with β-blockers.[93–95]

SELECTIVE I_f INHIBITORS IN REGIONAL MYOCARDIAL ISCHEMIA

Awareness that β-blockade not only reduces heart rate, but also the myocardial inotropic state, and unmasks α-adrenergic coronary vasoconstriction, has prompted the development of selective I_f inhibitors. Such agents are chemically distinct compounds, and the first drug that was advocated as a selective bradycardic agent was the clonidine derivative alinidine, in the early 1980s. Development of selective I_f inhibitors coincided with the detection of the sinoatrial pacemaker I_f current by DiFrancesco *et al*.[96,97]

The I_f current subsequently became the target of all selective bradycardic agents, including alinidine, the benzazepinones ULFS-49 and ivabradine, and others.[98–100] In conscious, chronically instrumented dogs with a coronary stenosis, alinidine reduced heart rate both at rest and during treadmill exercise. The ischemic contractile dysfunction that developed during exercise was attenuated, but this was at the expense of a significant negative inotropic effect, both at rest and during exercise.[101] Furthermore, in anesthetized pigs, alinidine decreased heart rate, caused a favorable redistribution of myocardial blood flow into the post-stenotic subendocardium and attenuated ischemic contractile dysfunction, but again at the expense of a negative inotropic action.[102]

ULFS-49 also decreased heart rate, both at rest and during exercise, in conscious, chronically instrumented dogs with a coronary stenosis. In consequence, post-stenotic subendocardial blood flow was improved[60] and ischemic contractile dysfunction attenuated; these beneficial effects were achieved in the absence of negative inotropic actions.[60,103] Despite its favorable anti-ischemic profile,

ULFS-49 resulted in frequent adverse events and was never developed further for clinical use.

The only currently available, selective bradycardic agent that has approval for clinical use is ivabradine (S 16257). Ivabradine in conscious, chronically instrumented dogs, causes a dose-dependent reduction in heart rate at rest and during exercise, and – in contrast to propranolol – exerts its effects without a negative inotropic action; in addition, ivabradine only slightly attenuates the epicardial coronary artery diameter increase during exercise, whereas propranolol actually reduces epicardial diameter, thus unmasking α-adrenergic coronary vasoconstriction (*Figure 4*).[104] Accordingly, ivabradine prolongs diastolic duration (thereby increasing perfusion) and reduces myocardial oxygen consumption (demand).[105,106] In chronically instrumented dogs with a coronary stenosis, ivabradine reduced heart rate at rest and during treadmill exercise, and improved post-stenotic subendocardial blood flow and contractile function; these beneficial effects during exercise-induced ischemia were followed by attenuation of post-ischemic contractile dysfunction (i.e. stunning), and attenuation of both ischemic and post-ischemic contractile function was lost when the reduction in heart rate was eliminated by atrial pacing. In contrast, β-blockade with atenolol also attenuated ischemic contractile dysfunction, but not post-ischemic stunning; atenolol also reduced non-ischemic wall function.[107,108] The attenuation by ivabradine of ischemic contractile dysfunction with reduced heart rate was confirmed in conscious pigs during treadmill exercise; such pigs also displayed less ST segment shift, similar to the effects of propranolol but without its negative inotropic action.[109] Apparently, in the animal experiment, ivabradine fulfilled all criteria for selectively decreasing heart rate without a negative inotropic action and without unmasking α-adrenergic coronary vasoconstriction. The effects of ivabradine on the flow–function relationship (perfusion–contraction match) and on infarct size during more prolonged ischemia have not been determined.

Recently, initial clinical data in patients with chronic stable angina have became available. In a double-blinded, placebo-controlled prospective trial, patients receiving ivabradine had prolonged time to 1-mm ST segment depression (*Figure 5*) and angina during exercise testing during 3 months of use, without any rebound following drug withdrawal.[110] In a rat model of post-myocardial infarction remodeling and heart failure, ivabradine reduced end-systolic, but not end-diastolic LV volume, thus increasing stroke volume and preserving cardiac output.[111] Furthermore, in patients with LV dysfunction, ivabradine reduced heart rate without an appreciable negative inotropic effect.[112]

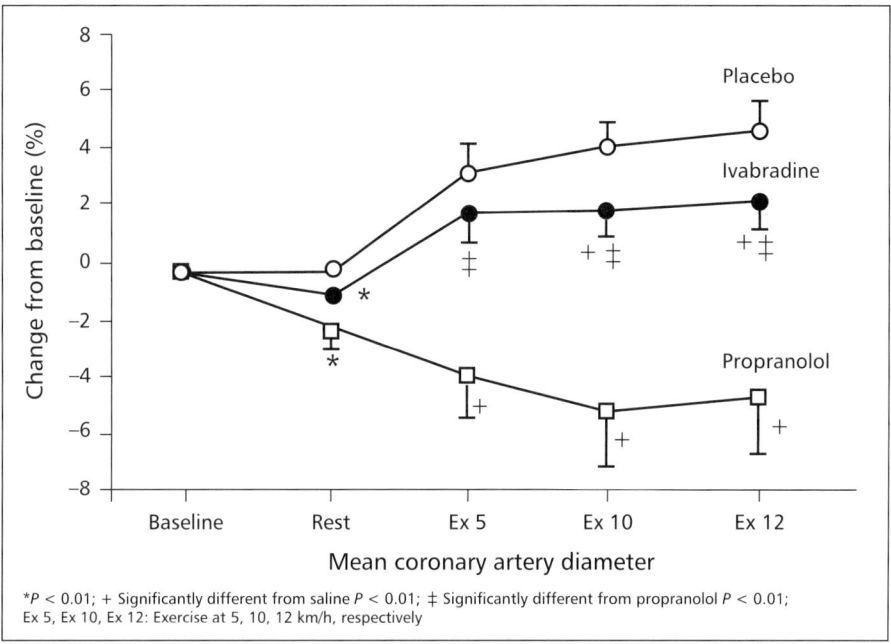

Figure 4 Increases in epicardial coronary artery diameter with increasing intensity of exercise with placebo (open circles) are only slightly attenuated with ivabradine (closed circles), whereas with propranolol (open squares) epicardial coronary artery diameter is decreased. From Simon et al.[104]

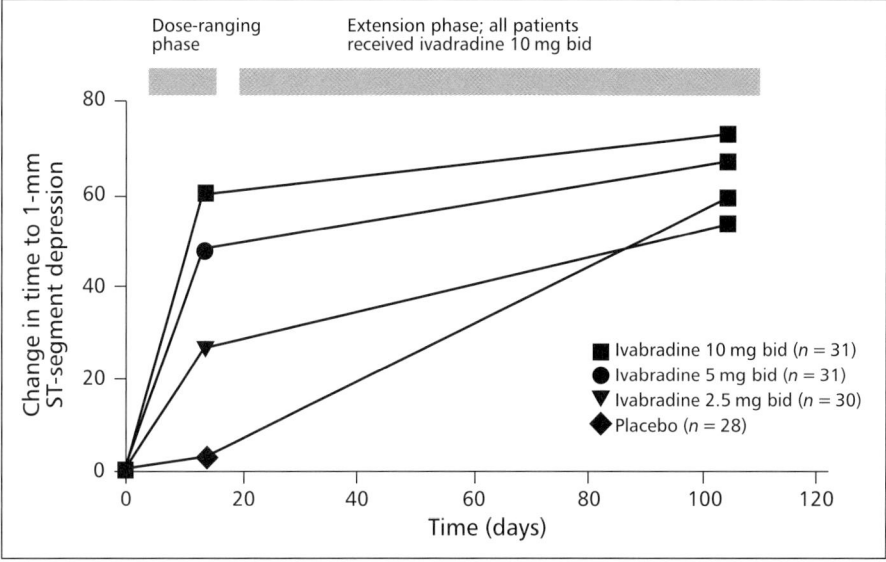

Figure 5 Changes in time to 1-mm ST-segment depression during exercise in patients with chronic stable angina. From Borer et al.[110]

In conclusion, increases in heart rate are of major importance in precipitating myocardial ischemia, predominantly through an unfavorable blood flow redistribution away from the ischemic subendocardium. Accordingly, selective reduction of heart rate attenuates the reductions in regional myocardial blood flow and contractile function, though importantly, not at the expense of a negative inotropic action or unmasked α-adrenergic coronary vasoconstriction.

REFERENCES

1. Hearse DJ. Myocardial ischemia: can we agree on a definition for the 21st century? *Cardiovasc Res*. 1994;28:1737–1744.

2. Heusch G, Schulz R. Perfusion–contraction match and mismatch. *Basic Res Cardiol*. 2001;96:1–10.

3. Heymann MA, Payne BD, Hoffman JIE, Rudolph AM. Blood flow measurements with radionuclide-labeled particles. *Prog Cardiovasc Dis*. 1977;20:55–78.

4. Bassingthwaighte JB, King RB, Roger SA. Fractal nature of regional myocardial blood flow heterogeneity. *Circ Res*. 1989;65:578–590.

5. Bassingthwaighte JB, Malone MA, Moffett TC, et al. Validity of microsphere depositions for regional myocardial flows. *Am J Physiol Heart Circ Physiol*. 1987;253:H184–H193.

6. Austin RE, Aldea GS, Coggins DL, et al. Profound spatial heterogeneity of coronary reserve. Discordance between patterns of resting and maximal myocardial blood flow. *Circ Res*. 1990;67:319–331.

7. Franzen D, Conway RS, Zhang H, et al. Spatial heterogeneity of local blood flow and metabolic content in dog hearts. *Am J Physiol Heart Circ Physiol*. 1988;254:H344–H353.

8. Schwanke U, Deussen A, Heusch G, Schipke JD. Heterogeneity of local myocardial flow and oxidative metabolism. *Am J Physiol Heart Circ Physiol*. 2000;279:H1029–H1035.

9. Sonntag M, Deussen A, Schultz J, et al. Spatial heterogeneity of blood flow in the dog heart. I. Glucose uptake, free adenosine and oxidative/glycolytic enzyme activity. *Pflügers Arch*. 1996;432:439–450.

10. Decking UKM, Skwirba S, Zimmermann MF, et al. Spatial heterogeneity of energy turnover in the heart. *Pflügers Arch*. 2001;441:663–673.

11. Laussmann T, Janosi RA, Fingas CD, et al. Myocardial proteome analysis reveals reduced NOS inhibition and enhanced glycolytic capacity in areas of low local blood flow. *Faseb J*. 2002;16:628–630.

12. Heusch G. Hibernating myocardium. Physiol Rev. 1998;78:1055–1085.

13. Kowallik P, Schulz R, Guth BD, et al. Measurement of regional myocardial blood flow with multiple colored microspheres. *Circulation*. 1991;83:974–982.

14. Bonow RO. Identification of viable myocardium. *Circulation*. 1996;94:2674–2680.

15. Camici PG, Gropler RJ, Jones T, et al. The impact of myocardial blood flow quantitation with PET on the understanding of cardiac diseases. *Eur Heart J*. 1996;17:25–34.

16. Schelbert HR. Positron emission tomography for the assessment of myocardial viability. *Circulation*. 1991;84 (Suppl I):I-122–I-131.

17. Sun KT, Czernin J, Krivokapich J, et al. Effects of dobutamine stimulation on myocardial blood flow, glucose metabolism, and wall motion in normal and dysfunctional myocardium. *Circulation*. 1996;94:3146–3154.

18. Marinho NVS, Keogh BE, Costa DC, et al. Pathophysiology of chronic left ventricular dysfunction. New insights from the measurement of absolute myocardial blood flow and glucose utilization. *Circulation*. 1996;93:737–744.

19. Gallagher KP, Osakada G, Matsuzaki M, et al. Nonuniformity of inner and outer systolic wall thickening in conscious dogs. *Am J Physiol Heart Circ Physiol*. 1985;249:H241–H248.

20. Sasayama S, Franklin D, Ross J Jr, et al. Dynamic changes in left ventricular wall thickness and their use in analyzing cardiac function in the conscious dog. *Am J Cardiol*. 1976;38:870–879.

21. Theroux P, Franklin D, Ross J Jr, Kemper WS. Regional myocardial function during acute coronary artery occlusion and its modification by pharmacological agents in the dog. *Circ Res*. 1974;35:896–908.

22. Theroux P, Ross J Jr, Franklin D, et al. Regional myocardial function in the conscious dog during acute coronary occlusion and responses to morphine, propranolol, nitroglycerin, and lidocaine. *Circulation*. 1976;53:302–314.

23. LeWinter MM, Kent RS, Kroener JM, et al. Regional differences in myocardial performance in the left ventricle of the dog. *Circ Res*. 1975;37:191–199.

24. Lew WYW, LeWinter MM. Regional comparison of midwall segment and area shortening in the canine left ventricle. *Circ Res*. 1986;58:678–691.

25. Gallagher KP, Osakada G, Hess OM, et al. Subepicardial segmental function during coronary stenosis and the role of myocardial fiber orientation. *Circ Res*. 1982;50:352–359.

26. Sabbah HN, Marzilli M, Stein PD. The relative role of subendocardium and subepicardium in left ventricular mechanics. *Am J Physiol Heart Circ Physiol*. 1981;240:H920–H926.

27. Waldman LK, Nosan D, Villarreal F, Covell JW. Relation between transmural deformation and local myofiber direction in canine left ventricle. *Circ Res*. 1988;63:550–562.

28. Waldman LK, Fung YC, Covell JW. Transmural myocardial deformation in the canine left ventricle. *Circ Res*. 1985;57:152–163.

29. Gayheart PA, Vinten-Johansen J, Johnston WE, et al. Oxygen requirements of the dyskinetic myocardial segment. *Am J Physiol Heart Circ Physiol*. 1989;257: H1184–H1191.

30. Downing SE. Wall tension and myocardial dysfunction after ischemia and reperfusion. *Am J Physiol Heart Circ Physiol*. 1993;264:H386–H393.

31. Chiu WC, Kedem J, Scholz PM, Weiss HR. Regional asynchrony of segmental contraction may explain the "oxygen consumption paradox" in stunned myocardium. *Basic Res Cardiol*. 1994;89:149–162.

32. Bassenge E, Heusch G. Endothelial and neuro-humoral control of coronary blood flow in health and disease. *Rev Physiol Biochem Pharmacol*. 1990;116:77-165.

33. Feigl EO. Coronary physiology. *Physiol Rev*. 1983;63:1–205.

34. Ross J Jr. Myocardial perfusion–contraction matching. Implications for coronary heart disease and hibernation. *Circulation*. 1991;83:1076–1083.

35. Schulz R, Guth BD, Heusch G. No effect of coronary perfusion on regional myocardial function within the autoregulatory range in pigs: Evidence against the Gregg phenomenon. *Circulation*. 1991;83:1390–1403.

36. Guth BD, Schulz R, Heusch G. Time course and mechanisms of contractile dysfunction during acute myocardial ischemia. *Circulation*. 1993;87 (Suppl. IV):IV-35–IV-42.

37. Vatner SF. Correlation between acute reductions in myocardial blood flow and function in conscious dogs. *Circ Res*. 1980;47:201–207.

38. Weintraub WS, Hattori S, Agarwal JB, et al. The relationship between myocardial blood flow and contraction by myocardial layer in the canine left ventricle during ischemia. *Circ Res*. 1981;48:430–438.

39. Gallagher KP, Matsuzaki M, Osakada G, et al. Effect of exercise on the relationship between myocardial blood flow and systolic wall thickening in dogs with acute coronary stenosis. *Circ Res*. 1983;52:716–729.

40. Gallagher KP, Matsuzaki M, Koziol JA, et al. Regional myocardial perfusion and wall thickening during ischemia in conscious dogs. *Am J Physiol Heart Circ Physiol*. 1984;247:H727–H738.

41. Indolfi C, Guth BD, Miura T, et al. Mechanisms of improved ischemic regional dysfunction by bradycardia. Studies on UL-FS 49 in swine. *Circulation*. 1989;80:983–993.

42. Indolfi C, Ross J Jr. The role of heart rate in myocardial ischemia and infarction: Implications of myocardial perfusion–contraction matching. *Prog Cardiovasc Dis*. 1993;36:61–74.

43. Buffington CW, Strum DP, Watanabe S. Regional oxygen consumption persists in dyskinetic canine myocardium. *J Cardiovasc Pharmacol*. 1994;24:37–44.

44. Heusch G, Post H, Michel MC, et al. Endogenous nitric oxide and myocardial adaptation to ischemia. *Circ Res*. 2000;87:146–152.

45. Kudej RK, Kim S-J, Shen Y-T, et al. Nitric oxide, an important regulator of perfusion–contraction matching in conscious pigs. *Am J Physiol Heart Circ Physiol*. 2000;279:H451–H456.

46. Sasayama S, Fujita M. Recent insights into coronary collateral circulation. *Circulation*. 1992;85:1197–1204.

47. Topol EJ, Ellis SG. Coronary collaterals revisited. Accessory pathway to myocardial preservation during infarction. *Circulation*. 1991;83:1084–1086.

48. Heusch G, Yoshimoto N. Effects of heart rate and perfusion pressure on segmental coronary resistances and collateral perfusion. *Pflügers Arch*. 1983;397:284–289.

49. Ertl G, Simm F, Wichmann J, et al. The dependence of coronary collateral blood flow on regional vascular resistances. *Naunyn Schmiedebergs Arch Pharmacol*. 1979;308:265–272.

50. Seiler C, Fleisch M, Meier B. Direct intracoronary evidence of collateral steal in humans. *Circulation*. 1997;96:4261–4267.

51. Billinger M, Fleisch M, Eberli FR, et al. Collateral and collateral-adjacent hyperemic vascular resistance changes and the psilateral coronary flow reserve: Documentation of a mechanism causing coronary steal in patients with coronary artery disease. *Cardiovasc Res*. 2001;49:600–608.

52. Holmvang G, Fry S, Skopicki HA, et al. Relation between coronary "steal" and contractile function at rest in collateral-dependent myocardium of humans with ischemic heart disease. *Circulation*. 1999;99:2510–2516.

53. Kyriakides ZS, Kremastinos DT, Kolettis TM, et al. Acute endothelin-A receptor antagonism prevents normal reduction of myocardial ischemia on repeated balloon inflations during angioplasty. *Circulation*. 2000;102:1937–1943.

54. Rowe GG. Inequalities of myocardial perfusion in coronary artery disease ("coronary steal"). *Circulation*. 1970;42:193–194.

55. Guyton RA, McClenathan JH, Newman GE, Michaelis LL. Significance of subendocardial S-T segment elevation caused by coronary stenosis in the dog. Epicardial S-T segment depression, local ischemia and subsequent necrosis. *Am J Cardiol*. 1977;40:373–380.

56. Gallagher KP, Folts JD, Shebuski RJ, et al. Subepicardial vasodilator reserve in the presence of critical coronary stenosis in dogs. *Am J Cardiol*. 1980;46:67–73.

57. Guth BD, Schulz R, Heusch G. Pressure-flow characteristics in the right and left ventricular perfusion territories of the right coronary artery in swine. *Pflügers Arch*. 1991;419:622–628.

58. Heusch G, Guth BD, Seitelberger R, Ross Jr. J. Attenuation of exercise-induced myocardial ischemia in dogs with recruitment of coronary vasodilator reserve by nifedipine. *Circulation*. 1987;75:482–490.

59. Guth BD, Heusch G, Seitelberger R, Ross J Jr. Mechanism of beneficial effect of beta-adrenergic blockade on exercise-induced myocardial ischemia in conscious dogs. *Circ Res*. 1987;60:738–746.

60. Guth BD, Heusch G, Seitelberger R, Ross J Jr. Elimination of exercise-induced regional myocardial dysfunction by a bradycardic agent in dogs with chronic coronary stenosis. *Circulation*. 1987;75:661–669.

61. Baumgart D, Ehring T, Krajcar M, Heusch G. A proischemic action of nisoldipine: relationship to a decrease in perfusion pressure and comparison to dipyridamole. *Cardiovasc Res*. 1993;27:1254–1259.

62. Guth BD, White FC, Gallagher KP, Bloor CM. Decreased systolic wall thickening in myocardium adjacent to ischemic zones in conscious swine during brief coronary artery occlusion. *Am Heart J*. 1984;107:458–464.

63. Gallagher KP, Gerren RA, Stirling MC, et al. The distribution of functional impairment across the lateral border of acutely ischemic myocardium. *Circ Res*. 1986;58:570–583.

64. Gallagher KP, Gerren RA, Ning X-H, et al. The functional border zone in conscious dogs. *Circulation*. 1987;76:929–942.

65. Buda AJ, Shlafer M, Gallagher KP. Spatial and temporal characteristics of circumferential flow-function relations during acute myocardial ischemia in the conscious dog. *Am Heart J*. 1988;116:1514–1523.

66. Gallagher KP. Regional myocardial flow - function relationship in ischemia. In Heusch G, ed. Pathophysiology and Rational Pharmacotherapy of Myocardial Ischemia. Darmstadt, New York: Steinkopff, Springer, 1990.

67. Bogen DK, Rabinowitz SA, Needleman A, et al. An analysis of the mechanical disadvantage of myocardial infarction in the canine left ventricle. *Circ Res*. 1980;47:728–741.

68. Stirling MC, Choy M, McClanahan TB, et al. Effects of ischemia on epicardial segment shortening. *J Surg Res*. 1991;50:30–39.

69. Homans DC, Sublett E, Lindstrom P, et al. Subendocardial and subepicardial wall thickening during ischemia in exercising dogs. *Circulation*. 1988;78:1267–1276.

70. Deussen A, Heusch G. Einfluss einer akuten Myokardischaemie auf die haemodynamischen Parameter des Restmyokards. Herzmedizin. 1984;7:32–35.

71. Lew WYW, Chen Z, Guth BD, Covell JW. Mechanisms of augmented segment shortening in nonischemic areas during acute ischemia of the canine left ventricle. *Circ Res*. 1985;56:351–358.

72. Heusch G, Guth BD, Widmann T, et al. Ischemic myocardial dysfunction assessed by temporal Fourier transform of regional myocardial wall thickening. *Am Heart J*. 1987;113:116–124.

73. Buda AJ, Lefkowitz CA, Gallagher KP. Augmentation of regional function in nonischemic myocardium during coronary occlusion measured with two-dimensional echocardiography. *J Am Coll Cardiol*. 1990;16:175–180.

74. Grines CL, Topol EJ, Califf RM, et al. Prognostic implications and predictors of enhanced regional wall motion of the noninfarct zone after thrombolysis and angioplasty therapy after acute myocardial infarction. *Circulation*. 1989;80:245–253.

75. Gascho JA, Beller GA. Adverse effects of circumflex coronary artery occlusion on blood flow to remote myocardium supplied by stenosed left anterior descending coronary artery in anesthetized open-chest dogs. *Am Heart J*. 1987;113:679–683.

76. Hasenfuss G, Holubarsch C, Hermann HP, et al. Influence of the force-frequency relationship on haemodynamics and left ventricular function in patients with non-failing hearts and in patients with dilated cardiomyopathy. *Eur Heart J*. 1994;15:164–170.

77. Raff WK, Kosche F, Lochner W. Heart rate and extravascular component of coronary resistance. *Pflügers Arch*. 1971;323:241–249.

78. Raff WK, Kosche F, Lochner W. Extravascular coronary resistance and its relation to microcirculation. *Am J Cardiol*. 1972; 29: 598–603.

79. Ferro G, Duilio C, Spinelli L, et al. Relation between diastolic perfusion time and coronary artery stenosis during stress-induced myocardial ischemia. *Circulation*. 1995;92:342–347.

80. Heusch G, Yoshimoto N, Müller-Ruchholtz ER. Effects of heart rate on hemodynamic severity of coronary artery stenosis in the dog. *Basic Res Cardiol*. 1982;77:562–573.

81. Santamore WP, Bove AA, Carey RA. Tachycardia induced reduction in coronary blood flow distal to a stenosis. *Int J Cardiol*. 1982;2:23–37.

82. Matsuzaki M, Patritti J, Tajimi T, et al. Effects of β-blockade on regional myocardial flow and function during exercise. *Am J Physiol*. 1984;247:H52–H60.

83. Buck JD, Hardman HF, Warltier DC, Gross GJ. Changes in ischemic blood flow distribution and dynamic severity of a coronary stenosis induced by beta blockade in the canine heart. *Circulation*. 1981;64:708–715.

84. Baumgart D, Haude M, Goerge G, et al. Augmented α-adrenergic constriction of atherosclerotic human coronary arteries. *Circulation*. 1999;99:2090–2097.

85. Gregorini L, Marco J, Kozàkovà M, et al. Alpha-adrenergic blockade improves recovery of myocardial perfusion and function after coronary stenting in patients with acute myocardial infarction. *Circulation*. 1999;99:482–490.

86. Heusch G, Baumgart D, Camici P, et al. α-Adrenergic coronary vasoconstriction and myocardial ischemia in humans. *Circulation*. 2000;101:689–694.

87. Gregorini L, Marco J, Farah B, et al. Effects of selective α1- and α2-adrenergic blockade on coronary flow reserve after coronary stenting. *Circulation*. 2002;106:2901–2907.

88. Gillman MW, Kannel WB, Belanger A, D'Agostino RB. Influence of heart rate on mortality among persons with hypertension: The Framingham study. *Am Heart J*. 1993;125:1148–1154.

89. Shaper AG, Wannamethee G, Macfarlane PW, Walker M. Heart rate, ischemic heart disease and sudden cardiac death in middle-aged British men. *Br Heart J*. 1993;70:49–55.

90. Palatini P, Casiglia E, Julius S, Pessina AC. High heart rate. A risk factor for cardiovascular death in elderly men. *Arch Intern Med*. 1999;159:585–592.

91. Hjalmarson A, Gilpin EA, Kjekshus J, et al. Influence of heart rate on mortality after acute myocardial infarction. *Am J Cardiol*. 1990;65:547–553.

92. Zuanetti G, Mantini L, Hernandez-Bernal F, et al. Relevance of heart rate as a prognostic factor in patients with acute myocardial infarction: insights from the GISSI-2 study. *Eur Heart J*. 1998;19:F19–F26.

93. CIBIS Investigators and Committees. The cardiac insufficiency bisoprolol study II (CIBIS-II): a randomised trial. *Lancet*. 1999;353:9–13.

94. MERIT-HF Study Group. Effect of metoprolol CR/XL in chronic heart failure: Metoprolol CR/XL randomised intervention trial in congestive heart failure. *Lancet*. 1999;353:2001–2007.

95. Packer M, Coats AJS, Fowler MB, et al. Effect of carvedilol on survival in severe chronic heart failure. *N Engl J Med*. 2001;344:1652–1658.

96. DiFrancesco D, Ojeda C. Properties of the current if in the sino-atrial node of the rabb compared with those of the current iK, in purkinje fibres. *J Physiol*. 1980;308:353–367.

97. DiFrancesco D. A study of ionic nature of the pace-maker current in calf purkinje fibres. *J Physiol*. 1981;314:377–393.

98. Ogiwara Y, Furukawa Y, Akahane K, et al. Bradycardic effects of AQ-A 39 (falipamil) in situ and in isolated, blood–perfused dog hearts. Comparison with alinidine and verapamil. *Jpn Heart J*. 1988;29:849–861.

99. BoSmith RE, Briggs I, Sturgess NC. Inhibitory actions of ZENECA ZD7288 on whole-cell hyperpolarization activated inward current (If) in guinea-pig dissociated sinoatrial node cells. *Br J Pharmacol*. 1993;110:343–349.

100. Thollon C, Cambarrat C, Vian J, et al. Electrophysiological effects of S 16257, a novel sino-atrial node modulator, on rabbit and guinea-pig cardiac preparations: comparisons with UL-FS 49. *Br J Pharmacol*. 1994;110:37–42.

101. Krumpl G, Mayer N, Schneider W, Raberger G. Effects of alinidine exercise-induced regional contractile dysfunction in dogs. *Eur J Pharmacol*. 1986;130:37–46.

102. Schamhardt HC, Verdouw PD, Saxena PR. Improvement of perfusion and function of ischaemic porcine myocardium after reduction of heart rate by alinidine. *J Cardiovasc Pharmacol*. 1981;3:728–738.

103. Simoons ML, Hugenholtz PG. Haemodynamic effects of alinidine, a specific sinus node inhibitor, in patients with unstable angina or myocardial infarction. *Eur Heart J*. 1984;5:227–232.

104. van de Werf F, Janssens L, Brzostek T, et al. Short-term effects of early intravenous treatment with a beta-adrenergic blocking agent or a specific bradycardiac agent in patients with acute myocardial infarction receiving thrombolytic therapy. *J Am Coll Cardiol*. 1993;22:407–416.

105. Krumpl G, Schneider W, Raberger G. Can exercise-induced regional contractile dysfunction be prevented by selective bradycardic agents? *Naunyn-Schmiedeberg's Arch Pharmacol*. 1986;334:540–543.

106. Indolfi C, Guth BD, Miyazaki S, et al. Heart rate reduction improves myocardial ischemia in swine: role of interventricular blood flow redistribution. *Am J Physiol*. 1991;261:H910–H917.

107. Schulz R, Rose J, Skyschally A, Heusch G. Bradycardic agent UL-FS 49 attenuates ischemic regional dysfunction and reduces infarct size in swine: comparison with the b-blocker atenolol. *J Cardiovasc Pharmacol*. 1995;25:216–228.

108. Simon L, Ghaleh B, Puybasset L, et al. Coronary and hemodynamic effects of S 16257, a new bradycardic agent, in resting and exercising conscious dogs. *J Pharmacol Exp Ther*. 1995;275:659–666.

109. Colin P, Ghaleh B, Monnet X, et al. Effect of graded heart rate reduction with ivabradine on myocardial oxygen consumption and diastolic time in exercising dogs. *J Pharmacol Exp Ther*. 2004;308:236–240.

110. Colin P, Ghaleh B, Monnet X, et al. Contributions of heart rate and contractility to myocardial oxygen balance during exercise. *Am J Physiol Heart Circ Physiol*. 2003;284:H676–H682.

111. Monnet X, Ghaleh B, Colin P, et al. Effects of heart rate reduction with ivabradine on exercise induced myocardial ischemia and stunning. *J Pharmacol Exp Ther*. 2001;299:1133–1139.

112. Monnet X, Colin P, Ghaleh B, et al. Heart rate reduction during exercise-induced myocardial ischaemia and stunning. *Eur Heart J*. 2004;3:1–8.

113. Vilaine J-P, Bidouard J-P, Lesage L, et al. Anti-ischemic effects of ivabradine, a selective heart rate-reducing agent, in exercise-induced myocardial ischemia in pigs. *J Cardiovasc Pharmacol*. 2003;42:688–696.

114. Borer JS, Fox K, Jaillon P, Lerebours G. Antianginal and antiischemic effects of ivabradine, an If inhibitor, in stable angina. *Circulation*. 2003;107:817–823.

115. Mulder P, Barbier S, Chagraoui A, et al. Long-term heart rate reduction induced by the selective If current inhibitor ivabradine improves left ventricular function and intrinsic myocardial structure in congestive heart failure. *Circulation*. 2004;109:1674–1679.

116. Manz M, Reuter M, Lauck G, Omran H. A single intravenous dose of ivabradine, a novel If inhibitor, lowers heart rate but does not depress left ventricular function in patients with left ventricular dysfunction. *Cardiology*. 2003;100:149–155.

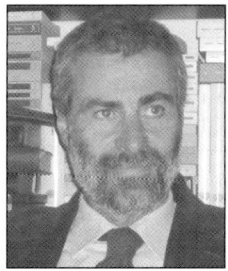

Antonio Zaza

4 Regulation of the sinoatrial pacemaker: selective I_f inhibition by ivabradine

Antonio Zaza, Marcella Rocchetti

Dipartimento di Biotecnologie e Bioscienze
Università Milano-Bicocca
20126 Milan, Italy
Tel: +39 02 64483307
Fax: +39 02 64483565
E-mail: antonio.zaza@unimib.it

INTRODUCTION

The purpose of this chapter is to discuss heart rate reduction by I_f inhibition, in terms of its basic mechanism and predicted impact on sinus-node physiology. Particular reference is made to ivabradine, the most recent I_f current inhibitor developed for clinical use. For illustrative purposes, mechanisms will be presented mainly through computer modeling of pacemaker activity and I_f behavior (OXSOFT HEART 4.8, Oxsoft Ltd, Oxford, UK). Nonetheless, the model used and the conclusions drawn are supported by experimental evidence, as specified in the references supplied.

A brief introduction to the basic concepts and language of cellular electrophysiology is provided for readers unacquainted with this discipline.

BASICS OF CELLULAR ELECTROPHYSIOLOGY

The electrical potential across the membrane of cardiac cells (membrane potential, E_m) is determined, at any instant, by a balance between charged molecules (ions) entering and leaving the cell through "ion channels". "Inward" and "outward" currents are generated by ions flowing into and out of the cell, respectively. Most cardiac currents are supported by positively charged ions (cations), which are moved through selective channels by gradients of concentration and charge that provide the "driving force" for the current. Thus, to generate a current, two conditions are needed: (1) an open channel and (2) a driving force for the ion to which the channel is permeable. Each current (I_K, I_f, etc.) is supported by the activity of many "single-channel" units, homogeneous for their selectivity and gating properties.

Channels are opened/closed by changes in membrane potential or by chemical signals. Some channels (e.g. those of I_{Na}, I_{Ca}, I_K) are opened when the membrane potential becomes more positive (depolarization), and others when it becomes more negative (repolarization or hyperpolarization) (e.g. those of I_{K1} and I_f). The fraction of total channel units of a given type (eg Ca^{2+} channels) open at each point in time is defined as the "open probability" (P_o) of the channel. The larger the P_o, the larger the "conductance" value of the current (the current per unit driving force value).

Ions are unevenly distributed across the membrane, partly due to the action of ion pumps – this results in ion concentration gradients and electrical charge gradients. Concentration and charge gradients have opposite directions and, when they balance each other (equilibrium), the net flow of ion is null. Equilibrium occurs at a membrane potential value called the "equilibrium potential", which is specific for each ion (E_K for K$^+$, E_{Na} for Na$^+$, etc.). The driving force for an ion is given by the difference between membrane potential and the ion's equilibrium potential. A current is inward if its driving force is negative (e.g. $E_m - E_K < 0$), and outward if the driving force is positive. Thus, each ion current reverses its direction at a membrane potential value called the "reversal potential" of the current. The reversal potential for a current carried by a single ion species is equal to the equilibrium potential of that ion; if the current is carried by different ions, its reversal potential is between their respective equilibrium potentials.

In living cells, the equilibrium potential of K$^+$ is negative (about –95 mV). Thus, when K$^+$ channels open, K$^+$ leaves the cell (outward current) and makes the inner side of the membrane negative (repolarization). Na$^+$ and Ca^{2+} ions have positive equilibrium potentials (above +70 mV); thus, opening of channels permeable to either of these ions generates an inward current, which leads to membrane depolarization.

Quiescent myocytes have a negative membrane potential (about –80 mV), mostly maintained by a large K$^+$ selective current (I_{K1}) in balance with a smaller background inward current (I_b), carried by voltage-insensitive Na$^+$ and Ca^{2+} channels.

To summarize, at rest, a membrane is polarized (negative inside); opening of Na$^+$ or Ca^{2+} channels (I_{Na}, I_{Ca}) depolarizes it, and opening of K$^+$ channels (I_K) brings the membrane potential back to the resting value (repolarization). The cardiac electrical cycle is, in essence, a sequence of changes in membrane conductance for specific ions. In this sequence, membrane potential changes are, at the same time, the result and cause of channel opening/closure. This provides the basis for auto-regenerative membrane depolarization, which is initiated once the membrane is depolarized to the "threshold potential" for Na$^+$ or Ca^{2+} channel opening.

In most cases, channel opening follows the change in membrane potential with a definite time course, which can be very rapid (µs for I_{Na} and I_{Ca}) or slow (from tens to hundreds of ms). Ion currents behaving in this way are said to be "time-dependent".

PACEMAKER MECHANISMS IN CARDIAC CELLS

The heart contains "automatic" cells, able to generate action potentials independently of other excitation sources, and non-automatic cells (e.g. ventricular myocytes). Pacemaker function is exerted by those automatic cells that beat at the fastest rate and are able to entrain all the remaining (follower) cells. Hence, automaticity and the ability to efficiently excite neighboring myocardium (generator properties) are both essential features of a pacemaker.

Automaticity

Automaticity results from an intrinsic tendency of membrane potential to oscillate, a sort of instability. When an oscillation achieves the threshold for excitation, an action potential ensues, which, in turn, sets the conditions for the following oscillation.

At an embryonic stage, all cardiac cells, including the precursors of atrial and ventricular myocardium, are endowed with automatic activity. Development into mature atrial or ventricular phenotypes includes loss of automaticity; this is associated with the appearance of I_{K1},[1] whose properties are ideally suited to stabilize the membrane potential at a constant value, negative to the action potential excitation threshold. Thus, loss of automaticity, rather than its presence, might be viewed as a functional specialization. This view is the conceptual basis for the recent proposal to generate artificial "biological" pacemakers by suppressing transcription of I_{K1} channels in localized areas of the ventricles.[2]

If lack of automaticity is afforded by I_{K1} expression, what is the mechanism for non-specific automaticity? Once I_{K1} is removed, background inward current (I_b)[3] depolarizes the membrane above the threshold for I_{Ca}, and triggers an action potential (including I_K activation). Following repolarization, I_K slowly decays; thus, the current balance turns again in favor of I_b and the cycle is restarted.[4] Moreover, recent work suggests that cytosolic Ca^{2+} oscillators may also contribute to cardiac automaticity through an interplay with Ca^{2+}-sensitive membrane currents.[5,6] To summarize, even if a single pacemaker mechanism may prevail under specific conditions, many are also available in cardiac tissues other than the sinoatrial (SA) node.

Generator properties

Provided cells are electrically connected by gap junctions, propagation of excitation depends on the availability of sufficient positive intracellular charge in one cell, which is transferred to neighboring cells, bringing their membranes to the excitation threshold. In ventricular cells, this charge is provided by the fast Na$^+$ current (I_{Na}); in SA and atrioventricular (AV) nodal cells, I_{Na} is absent and is replaced by the Ca^{2+} current I_{CaL}. Thus, in the SA and AV nodes, propagation is said to be Ca^{2+}-dependent.

PACEMAKER MECHANISMS IN THE SINOATRIAL NODE

Under normal conditions, the SA node acts as the pacemaking structure of the heart. I_{K1} is not expressed in SA node myocytes, which is probably the key feature that endows them with automaticity. Nonetheless, SA electrical activity also includes specificities, not shared by other cell types, which afford functional advantages in terms of stabilization of the oscillator and fine modulation of its rate. Indeed, a current named I_f is selectively expressed in the SA node and, to a lesser extent, in other tissues serving as subsidiary pacemakers (AV node and Purkinje). I_f is ideally suited to support automaticity:[7-11]

(1) f-channels are closed by positive potentials and opened by negative potentials (hyperpolarization-activated current).

(2) I_f current is time-dependent, i.e. once the membrane potential is changed, its channels open (or close) over a certain amount of time. Membrane hyperpolarization increases I_f activation (opening) rate, and depolarization increases I_f deactivation (closing) rate.

(3) f-channels are permeable to both Na$^+$ and K$^+$; I_f reversal potential (E_f) is close to –20 mV. Thus, membrane potential is negative to E_f in diastole and becomes positive to it during the action potential. Provided f-channels are open, I_f current is inward during diastole and outward during the action potential.

(4) I_f current is strongly increased by adrenergic activation (β1 receptors) and depressed by vagal activation (M2 receptors). Channel modulation is carried out directly by cytosolic cAMP, whose concentration is increased by β1 and decreased by M2 receptors. The short time required for cAMP action on the channel (less than a cardiac cycle) allows autonomic control of heart rate on a beat-to-beat basis.

The contribution of I_f current to the various phases of the SA cycle is illustrated by the model reconstruction shown in *Figure 1*.

(1) When the repolarization process causes the membrane potential to become sufficiently negative (threshold at about $-40\,\text{mV}$), I_f slowly turns on (P_o increases); this results in inward current (*Figure 1B*), which progressively depolarizes the membrane potential toward the threshold for the activation of I_{Ca}, which then turns on and supports the next action potential. A larger I_f leads to steeper diastolic depolarization and a more rapid sinus rate.

(2) When the next action potential ensues (dashed line), a portion of the f-channels remain open ($P_o > 0$ in *Figure 1C*). The membrane potential becomes rapidly positive to E_f (driving force becomes positive in *Figure 1D*) and I_f current switches to the outward direction (*Figure 1B*). However, during the action potential, I_f is short-lived because its channels are rapidly closed by depolarization (P_o declines).

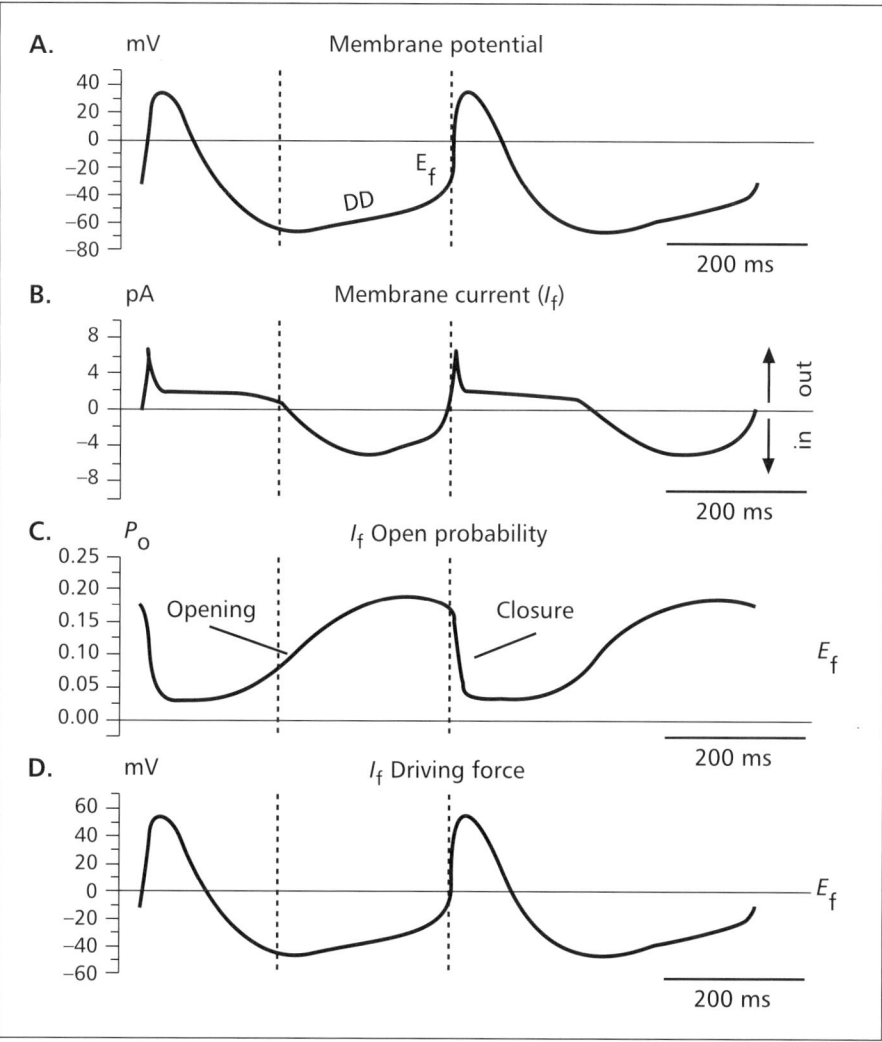

Figure 1 Time course of I_f current and the underlying f-channel function during a sinoatrial pacemaker cycle. Traces in panels A–D are time-aligned; the dashed lines encompass the diastolic interval. A. Pacemaker activity is generated by diastolic depolarization (DD). B. I_f flows in the inward direction (in) during diastolic depolarization and turns briefly outward (out) during the action potential upstroke. C. The open probability of f-channels (P_o) slowly increases during the diastole and rapidly declines during the action potential. Persistence of $P_o > 0$ during membrane depolarization allows I_f to flow in the outward direction. D. The driving force for I_f is negative during diastole, positive during the action potential and null when membrane potential equals the I_f reversal potential (E_f)

Some of the I_f current features act as fail-safe mechanisms, which limit the range of variability of the cardiac cycle[12] and assist in its fine modulation.

(1) Under normal conditions, I_f is largely redundant; only a small proportion of total f-channels (P_o in *Figure 1C*) activate during a normal diastolic interval. Since activation is slow, prolongation of the diastolic interval recruits more I_f, thus preventing further prolongation. This may protect pacemaker function from partial I_f blockade (*Figure 2*) and changes in the threshold of excitation (e.g. by Ca^{2+} channel blockers), etc.

(2) Other currents beside I_f flow during the diastolic interval, and the rate of diastolic depolarization depends on their net balance. In addition to inhibiting I_f current, acetylcholine activates a large K^+ current (I_{KACh}), which hyperpolarizes the membrane potential and tends to suppress pacemaker activity.[13] However, the latter is readily recovered by the hyperpolarization-induced increase in I_f, which acts as a very efficient buffer. Indeed, model simulation suggests that if acetylcholine action was limited to I_{KACh} activation, unphysiologically high concentrations would be required to modulate pacemaker rate. On the other hand, if I_f were entirely removed, pacemaker rate would be modulated by acetylcholine in a narrower range of concentrations, with instability occurring at higher concentrations. This is illustrated in *Figure 3*, in which modulation by acetylcholine (acting on I_f and I_{KACh}) was applied to pacemaking based on I_f or I_b (I_f made negligible). Thus, I_f may be pivotal for a graded response of sinus rate to vagal activation.

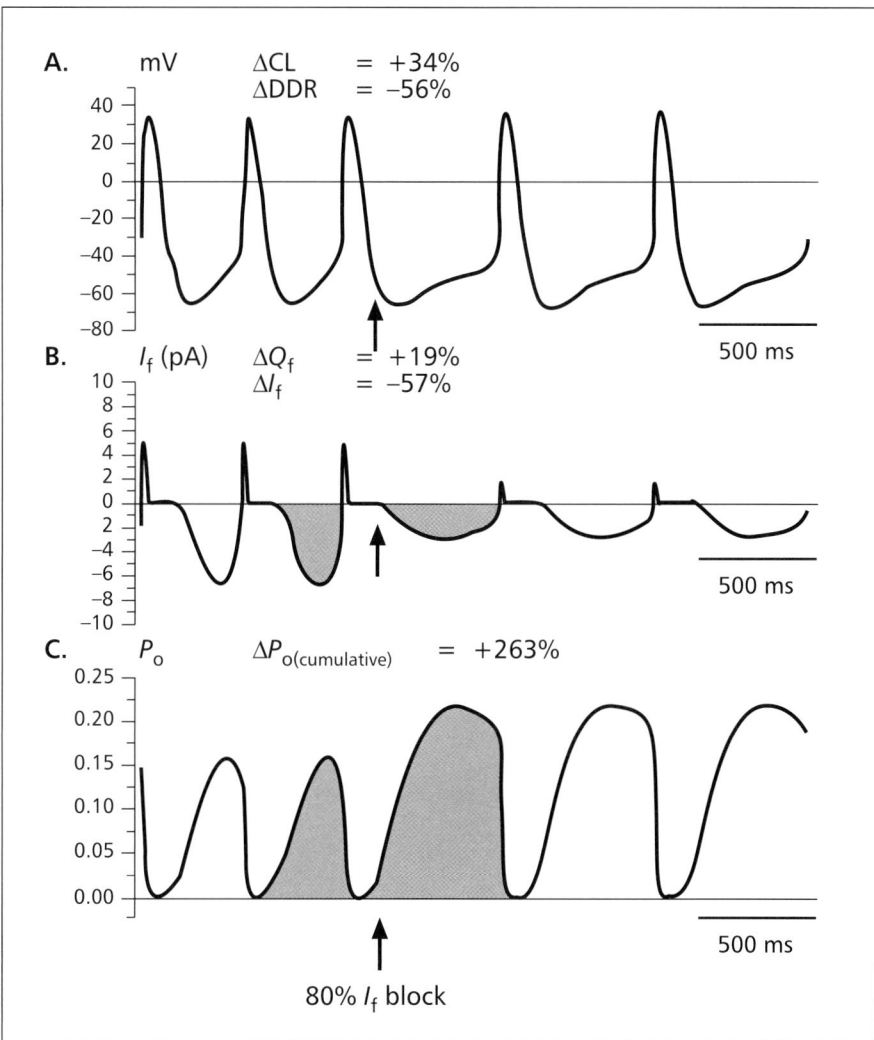

Figure 2 Mechanism of I_f "functional reserve." The model is set to produce I_f-dependent pacemaking (i.e. 100% I_f block causes arrest). 80% of f-channels were inhibited at the instant marked by the arrows, which increased pacemaker cycle length (CL) by 34% (A) and reduced inward charge flow through I_f (Q_f) by only 19%. The apparent discrepancy between the extent of I_f inhibition and its effect on CL and Q_f is due to the increase in the P_o of unblocked f-channels (cumulative P_o increased by 263%), a consequence of the longer diastolic interval (C). Shaded areas in the I_f and P_o traces correspond to Q_f and cumulative P_o, respectively

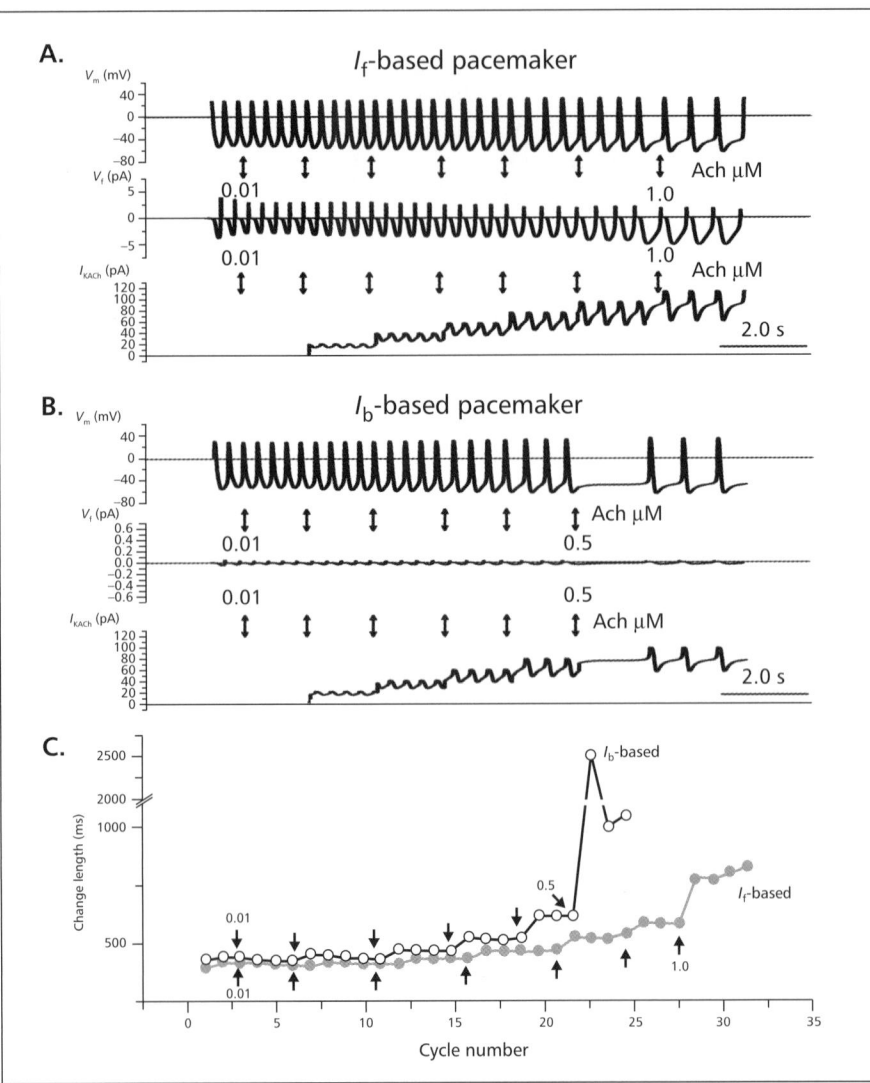

Figure 3 Response of I_f- and I_b-based pacemaking to acetylcholine ([ACh] 0.01–1.0 µm). Concentration-dependent ACh effects are simulated according to references 10 and 13. Each panel shows membrane potential (upper trace), I_f (middle trace) and I_{KACh} (bottom trace); arrows mark progressive [ACh] increments. A. I_f-based pacemaker. The slowing effect of I_{KACh} activation is blunted by the hyperpolarization-induced increase in I_f, thus resulting in smooth regulation of pacemaker rate up to 1 µm ACh. B. I_b-based pacemaker. Steeper rate slowing occurs at low [ACh] due to unbalanced I_{KACh} activation; however, marked pacemaker instability already occurs at 0.5 µm ACh. C. Cycle length changes observed in the I_f-based and I_b-based models, respectively

I_f AS A SPECIFIC PHARMACOLOGICAL TARGET TO REDUCE HEART RATE

I_f involvement in physiological pacemaker function makes it an obvious target for pharmacological modulation of heart rate. It is interesting, therefore, to consider the potential advantages and drawbacks of I_f current inhibitors, compared with β-blockers and Ca^{2+} antagonists, the other tools currently available.

Within the heart, the only function exerted by I_f is pacemaking. Thus, I_f inhibition may reduce sinus rate without affecting contractility or impulse propagation. This is clearly different from the wide spectrum of effects of β-blockers, and can be seen as an advantage under many conditions. On the other hand, with the exception of the aspects secondary to tachycardia, I_f inhibitors will not reduce the impact of sympathetic activation on cardiac muscle.

A further advantage of targeting I_f is that the "generator" properties of the sinus node may be unaffected. Indeed, during the action potential upstroke, I_f current is outward (*Figure 1B*); therefore, even if only to a minor extent (1–2%), its inhibition would increase the net inward current entering the cell. This is clearly different from reducing the sinus rate by blocking I_{Ca} (as with Ca^{2+} antagonists), which is the major source of inward current in the node. SA conduction block is among the most frequent cause of pacemaker failure in the clinical setting, particularly in the elderly population. Thus, the theoretical advantage of targeting I_f, rather than Ca^{2+} channels, may be significant.

As discussed above, I_f has an important role in pacemaking; the question arises, therefore, of whether I_f current inhibition might compromise sinus function. Experimental evidence indicates that even substantial I_f inhibition does not lead to a dramatic decrease in pacemaking rate, and preserves the response to autonomic agonists.[14] Although compensation by other currents might contribute, model analysis shows that this would occur even if these were not available. In fact, under conditions in which 100% I_f blockade leads to complete pacemaker arrest (I_f-dependent pacemaking), 80% I_f inhibition is still compatible with a relatively small reduction in rate (*Figure 2*). Such an extraordinary "functional reserve" may actually be intrinsic to I_f and result from its fail-safe properties (described above). Additional functional reserve may be provided by a shift of the dominant pacemaker to regions, within the sinus node, with different sensitivity to inhibitory stimuli.[15] Thus, as long as it is incomplete, I_f

current inhibition is unlikely to compromise sinus-node function significantly. Nonetheless, a reduction of pacemaking functional reserve, proportional to the extent of I_f inhibition, is theoretically expected, and its practical relevance in the wide spectrum of conditions peculiar to the clinical setting remains to be established.

THE I_f INHIBITOR IVABRADINE AS A TOOL FOR HEART RATE REDUCTION

In terms of mechanism of action, the important features to be considered in selecting an I_f inhibitor for pure heart rate reduction are:

(1) Selectivity of action on I_f current with respect to other ion currents within the heart or in other tissues;

(2) Rate-dependency of block and interaction with neurotransmitters

Selectivity of action

Ivabradine has been shown to inhibit I_f in rabbit SA myocytes with 50% maximal effect at concentrations (EC$_{50}$) below 3 µm.[16,17] The concentration–response curve for I_f inhibition covered a rather wide range, with a threshold at 0.1 µm and saturation at >10 µm. The spontaneous rate of multicellular atrial preparations was decreased by ivabradine in the same range of concentrations.[18,19]

I_K inhibition causes proarrhythmic repolarization abnormalities (iatrogenic long-QT);[20] therefore, its absence within the therapeutic range of concentrations is of particular relevance. In rabbit SA myocytes, I_K was unaffected by ivabradine at the measured concentration of 3 µM. In guinea-pig ventricular muscle, paced at slow rate (1 Hz), 1 µM ivabradine marginally prolonged action potential duration (6%).[19]

Slight inhibition of L-type Ca^{2+} currents (18%) was observed with 10 µm ivabradine in SA myocytes,[16] whereas no detectable blockade was recorded on T-type Ca^{2+} currents. The relative lack of effect on L-type Ca^{2+} current suggests an absence of negative inotropy induced by ivabradine.[16] A decrease in the maximum velocity of action potential upstroke, suggesting I_{Na} block, occurred in ventricular muscle with a threshold at 5 µm.[18]

Taken together, the results of *in vitro* studies show that the effect of ivabradine is selective throughout two-thirds of its I_f inhibition curve; other currents become marginally affected at concentrations at which I_f inhibition saturates. With such a profile, ivabradine is currently the most selective I_f inhibitor. Extrapolation of the concentration-dependency of effects observed *in vitro* to the clinical setting would require knowledge of intramyocardial drug concentrations. These cannot be directly measured in man, and are hardly predictable. Nonetheless, according to the clinical studies available to date, ivabradine regimens are associated with significant negative chronotropy (12–18% reduction in resting heart rate), and preservation of QTc interval, conduction time and myocardial contractility.[21,22]

An isoform of the f-channel protein (HCN1) is expressed in retinal photoreceptors,[23] and is responsible for the inhibitory effect that these cells exert on the retinal circuit during darkness. Blockade of this channel accounts for reversible visual side-effects (persistent images, phosphenes), which are induced by all I_f inhibitors, including ivabradine, at high dosages.[24]

Rate-dependency of block and interaction with neural stimulation

Experimental studies have demonstrated that the effect of ivabradine increases as the interval between I_f activations is shortened (rate-dependent inhibition).[17] Accordingly, ivabradine-induced bradycardia is more pronounced during exercise in dogs.[25] This is a practically relevant feature of the action of ivabradine, and it is interesting to consider whether it can be interpreted based on the present knowledge on ivabradine interaction with f-channels.

Ivabradine is a charged molecule and binds to a site within the channel pore, which can be reached only from the cytoplasmic side.[16] Access to the binding site is possible only when the channel is open; therefore, ivabradine is said to be an "open" channel inhibitor.[17] With this in mind, one would expect ivabradine I_f current inhibition to develop mainly during the diastolic interval (when I_f is turned on). However, ivabradine appears to be removed from its binding site by the current flowing in the inward direction; thus, while opening of the f-channels during diastole is necessary to allow ivabradine to enter, the extent of I_f inhibition that can develop during this phase is limited. Conversely, ivabradine I_f inhibition is favored if the current flows in the outward direction,[17] a condition achieved only during the very early portion of the action potential, when f-channels are still open (*Figures 1B and 1C*). Since outward I_f current is short-lived, only a small proportion of f-channels are blocked during a single action potential, and some of them are unblocked when channels reopen during the following diastole.

If ivabradine inhibition develops during outward flow and wanes during inward I_f flow, the overall extent of I_f inhibition should depend on the balance between outward (Q_{out}) and inward (Q_{in}) charge flow occurring in each cycle. The question then turns to how this balance can be affected by an increase in pacemaker rate. Since, under physiological conditions, this is generally due to a change in the autonomic balance, it is practical to consider how the Q_{out}/Q_{in} ratio would be affected by β-adrenergically induced tachycardia. In *Figure 4*, this condition is reproduced by changes in all the currents known to be affected by β-receptors (I_{Ca}, I_K, I_f).[10,26] As shown in the Figure, an adrenergically induced increase in rate (CL shortening) is expected to increase the Q_{out}/Q_{in} ratio. This is partly due to shortening of the time spent in diastole, but it also depends on receptor-induced changes in I_f properties.

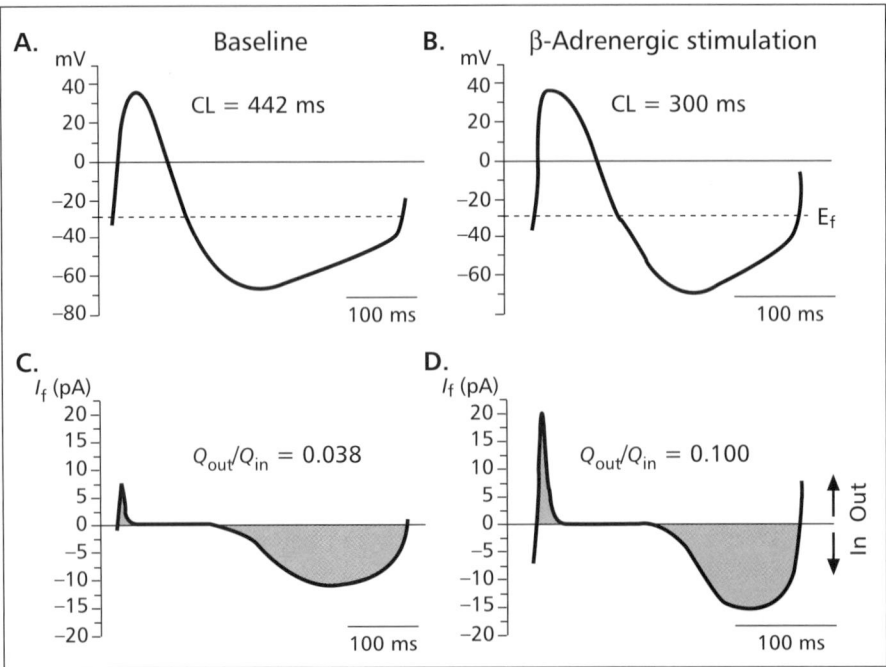

Figure 4 Effect of β-adrenergic stimulation on outward (out) and inward (in) charge flow (Q) through I_f. Q corresponds to the shaded areas under outward (Q_{out}) and inward (Q_{in}) current. β-Adrenergic effects are simulated according to reference 10. Adrenergically induced shortening of CL (A, B) is associated with a sharp increase in the Q_{out}/Q_{in} ratio (C, D)

According to the above, an increase in the Q_{out}/Q_{in} ratio during adrenergically induced tachycardia predicts that drug effects may be increased during exercise, as was indeed observed in dogs.[25] Therefore, the report that, in humans, the absolute change in heart rate induced by ivabradine is similar at rest and during peak exercise[24] is unexpected, and its mechanistic interpretation may require additional information.

CONCLUSIONS

Selective inhibition of I_f current reduces heart rate without affecting other cardiac functions. Due to the presence of a considerable "functional reserve", even substantial I_f inhibition is unlikely to abolish pacemaker function completely. Ivabradine is currently the most selective I_f current inhibitor. The features of ivabradine-induced inhibition are such as to predict a stronger effect during tachycardia, particularly if the latter results from sympathetic activation.

REFERENCES

1. Maltsev VA, Wobus AM, Rohwedel J, et al. Cardiomyocytes differentiated in vitro from embryonic stem cells developmentally express cardiac-specific genes and ionic currents. *Circ Res*. 1994;75:233–244.

2. Miake J, Marban E, Nuss HB. Biological pacemaker created by gene transfer. *Nature*. 2002;419:132–133.

3. Hagiwara N, Irisawa H, Kasanuki H, et al. Background current in sino-atrial node cells of the rabbit heart. *J Physiol*. 1992;448:53–72.

4. Irisawa H, Brown HF, Giles W. Cardiac pacemaking in the sinoatrial node. *Physiol Rev*. 1993;73:197–227.

5. Vinogradova TM, Zhou YY, Maltsev V, et al. Rhythmic ryanodine receptor Ca2+ releases during diastolic depolarization of sinoatrial pacemaker cells do not require membrane depolarization. *Circ Res*. 2004;94:802–809.

6. Lakatta EG, Maltsev VA, Bogdanov KY, et al. Cyclic variation of intracellular calcium: a critical factor for cardiac pacemaker cell dominance. *Circ Res*. 2003;92:e45–e50.

7. DiFrancesco D, Ferroni A, Mazzanti M, et al. Properties of the hyperpolarizing-activated current (if) in cells isolated from the rabbit sino-atrial node. *J Physiol*. 1986;377:61–88.

8. DiFrancesco D, Tortora P. Direct activation of cardiac pacemaker channels by intracellular cyclic AMP. *Nature*. 1991;351:145–147.

9. DiFrancesco D, Zaza A. The cardiac pacemaker current If. *J Cardiovasc Electrophysiol*. 2000;11:1289–1293. 1992;3:334–344.

10. Zaza A, Robinson RB, DiFrancesco D. Basal responses of the L-type Ca2+ and hyperpolarization-activated currents to autonomic agonists in the rabbit sinoatrial node. *J Physiol*. 1996;491:347–355.

11. Zaza A, Micheletti M, Brioschi A, et al. Ionic currents during sustained pacemaker activity in rabbit sino-atrial myocytes. *J Physiol*. 1997;505:677–688.

12. Noble D, Denyer JC, Brown HF, et al. Reciprocal role of the inward currents Ib,Na and If in controlling and stabilizing pacemaker frequency of rabbit sino-atrial node cells. *Proc R Soc Lond B*. 1992;250:199–207.

13. DiFrancesco D, Ducouret P, Robinson RB. Muscarinic modulation of cardiac rate at low acetylcholine concentrations. *Science*. 1989;243:669–671.

14. Boyett MR, Kodama I, Honjo H, et al. The role of the hyperpolarization-activated current and the muscarinic K+ current in the chronotropic effect of ACh on the sinoatrial node isolated from the rabbit. *J Physiol*. 1993;467:159P.

15. Boyett MR, Honjo H, Kodama I. The sinoatrial node, a heterogeneous pacemaker structure. *Cardiovasc Res*. 2000;47:658–687.

16. Bois P, Bescond J, Renaudon B, et al. Mode of action of bradycardic agent, S 16257, on ionic currents of rabbit sinoatrial node cells. *Br J Pharmacol*. 1996;118:1051–1057.

17. Bucchi A, Baruscotti M, DiFrancesco D. Current-dependent block of rabbit sino-atrial node I(f) channels by ivabradine. *J Gen Physiol*. 2002;120:1–13.

18. Perez O, Gay P, Franqueza L, et al. Effects of the two enantiomers, S-16257-2 and S-16260-2, of a new bradycardic agent on guinea-pig isolated cardiac preparations. *Br J Pharmacol*. 1995;115:787–794.

19. Thollon C, Cambarrat C, Vian J, et al. Electrophysiological effects of S 16257, a novel sino-atrial node modulator, on rabbit and guinea-pig cardiac preparations: comparison with UL-FS 49. *Br J Pharmacol*. 1994;112:37–42.

20. Moss AJ. The QT interval and torsade de pointes. *Drug Safety*. 1999;21(Suppl 1):5–10.

21. Camm AJ, Lau CP. Electrophysiological effects of a single intravenous administration of ivabradine (S 16257) in adult patients with normal baseline electrophysiology. *Drugs R D*. 2003;4:83–89.

22. Manz M, Reuter M, Lauck G, et al. A single intravenous dose of ivabradine, a novel I(f) inhibitor, lowers heart rate but does not depress left ventricular function in patients with left ventricular dysfunction. *Cardiology*. 2003;100:149–155.

23. Demontis GC, Moroni A, Gravante B, et al. Functional characterisation and subcellular localisation of HCN1 channels in rabbit retinal rod photoreceptors. *J Physiol*. 2002;542:89–97.

24. Borer JS, Fox K, Jaillon P, et al. Antianginal and antiischemic effects of ivabradine, an I(f) inhibitor, in stable angina: a randomized, double-blind, multicentered, placebo-controlled trial. *Circulation*. 2003;107:817–823.

25. Simon L, Ghaleh B, Puybasset L, et al. Coronary and hemodynamic effects of S 16257, a new bradycardic agent, in resting and exercising conscious dogs. *J Pharmacol Exp Ther*. 1995;275:659–666.

26. Noma A, Kotake H, Irisawa H. Slow inward current and its role mediating the chronotropic effect of epinephrine in the rabbit sinoatrial node. *Pflügers Arch*. 1980;388:1–9.

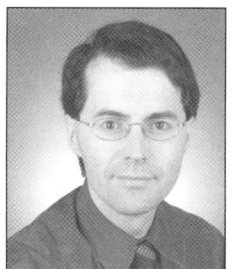

Jean-Claude Tardif

5 Clinical benefits of exclusive heart rate reduction in stable angina

Ariel Diaz, Jean-Claude Tardif

Montreal Heart Institute
5000 Belanger Street
Montreal, Canada, H1T 1C8
Tel: 514 376 3330, ext.3612
Fax: 514 593 2500
E-mail: jean-claude.tardif@icm-mhi.org

INTRODUCTION

Chronic stable angina is a common and disabling condition, affecting 30–40 000 per 1 million people in Europe and the US. Angina occurs when myocardial perfusion is insufficient to meet metabolic demand. Individuals with typical chronic stable angina usually have significant narrowing of at least one major epicardial vessel, and experience pain that is related to an increase in physical activity or psychological stress. Heart rate is one of the most important determinants of myocardial oxygen demand. A high heart rate induces or exacerbates myocardial ischemia and subsequent angina, since it both increases myocardial oxygen demand and decreases myocardial perfusion, the latter by shortening the duration of diastole.

Relieving the symptoms of angina and improving the quality of life and functional status of patients are integral components of the management of chronic stable angina.[1] β-Blockers are effective at reducing anginal symptoms, mainly by decreasing heart rate,[2] and are usually preferred as initial therapy in the absence of contraindications.[3] Despite the demonstrated safety and effectiveness of β-blockers, physician use and patient compliance may be somewhat limited by the side-effects of this class of agents, which include fatigue, sexual dysfunction, depression, cold extremities, light-headedness, gastrointestinal disturbances, bronchospasm and atrioventricular (AV) block.[4–7] β-blockade can also increase coronary resistance and limit exercise-induced increases in coronary arterial flow.[8,9] In addition, β-blockers can reduce left ventricular contractility.[10] Finally, this class of agents may have detrimental effects on carbohydrate and lipid metabolism.[11,12]

Ivabradine (Procoralan), a novel heart-rate-lowering agent, acts by selectively inhibiting the I_f current involved in the pacemaker activity of sinoatrial node cells.[13,14] I_f current is a mixed sodium–potassium inward current activated by hyperpolarization and modulated by the autonomic nervous system, and is one of the most important ionic currents for the regulation of pacemaker depolarization. Ivabradine has been shown to reduce heart rate at rest and during exercise in experimental animals[10,15–17] and healthy human volunteers.[18] In contrast to β-blockers, ivabradine does not have detrimental effects on coronary vasomotion or myocardial contractility in animals.[10,19] In addition, ivabradine does not appear to affect AV node and His-Purkinje conduction or ventricular repolarization.[20]

ANTI-ISCHEMIC AND ANTI-ANGINAL EFFECTS OF IVABRADINE

The anti-anginal and anti-ischemic effects of ivabradine were first investigated in a randomized, double-blind, multicenter, placebo-controlled clinical trial.[21] In this elegantly designed trial, 360 patients with a history of at least 3 months of chronic stable angina and documented coronary artery disease (diagnosed by angiography or indicated by previous myocardial infarction at least 3 months before randomization) were randomly assigned, after a washout period of anti-anginal medications, to receive one of three doses of ivabradine (2.5, 5 or 10 mg bid) or placebo for 2 weeks (*Figure 1*). This was followed by an open-label 2-month or 3-month extension phase, during which all patients received ivabradine 10 mg bid. Patients were then randomly assigned to continue on ivabradine 10 mg bid, or to withdraw to placebo for 1 week. The primary efficacy endpoints were the changes from baseline in time to 1-mm ST-segment depression and the time to limiting angina during bicycle exercise tolerance tests (ETTs) performed at troughs of drug activity.

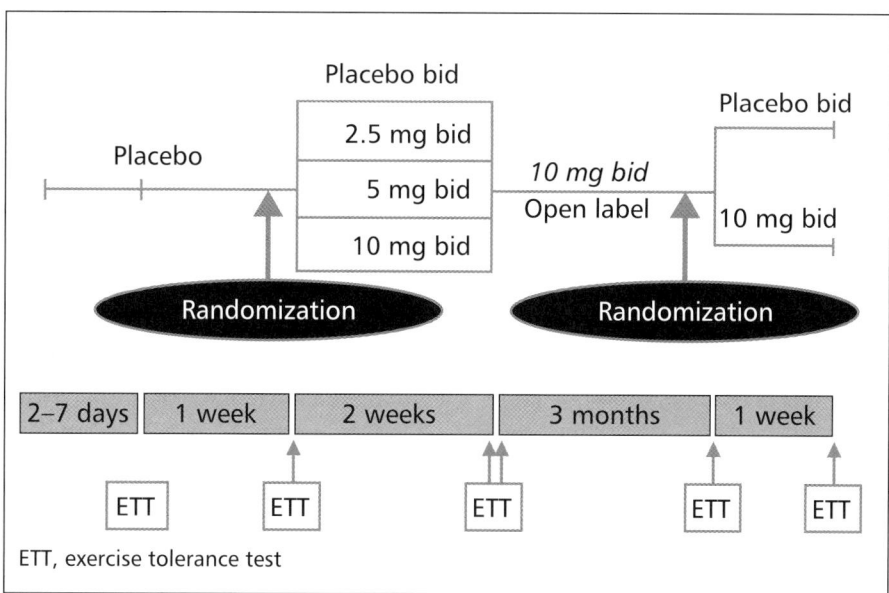

Figure 1 Design features of a multicenter, double-blind, placebo-controlled, dose-ranging study of ivabradine in 360 patients with documented coronary artery disease. From Borer et al.[21]

Between the start and end of the double-blind, dose-ranging phase, resting heart rate and maximal heart rate during exercise significantly decreased in all three active treatment groups, compared with placebo (*Figure* 2). Ivabradine 10 mg bid reduced both resting heart rate and maximal heart rate by 12–13 bpm ($P < 0.05$). Time to 1-mm ST-segment depression during ETTs improved with ivabradine treatment in a dose-related fashion, and the increase was significant in the 5 mg and 10 mg bid groups ($P < 0.05$, *Figure* 3). Time to limiting angina increased significantly with ivabradine, in comparison with placebo, in the 10-mg bid group (mean increase: 41 s, $P < 0.05$). Ivabradine-mediated improvements in time to 1-mm ST-segment depression and time to limiting angina in the double-blind phase were maintained in the open-label phase. In addition, angina attacks were reduced from a mean of approximately four attacks per week at baseline to < 1 attack per week at the end of the open-label extension ($P < 0.001$). During the double-blind, randomized withdrawal period, patients who were continued on ivabradine 10 mg bid maintained the benefits on heart rate, time to 1-mm ST-segment depression and time to limiting angina, whereas ETT parameters deteriorated in patients withdrawn to placebo (*Figure* 4). Importantly, no rebound phenomena were observed on treatment cessation. In summary, ivabradine demonstrated dose-dependent anti-ischemic and anti-anginal effects at the doses of 5 mg bid and 10 mg bid in this placebo-controlled study.[21]

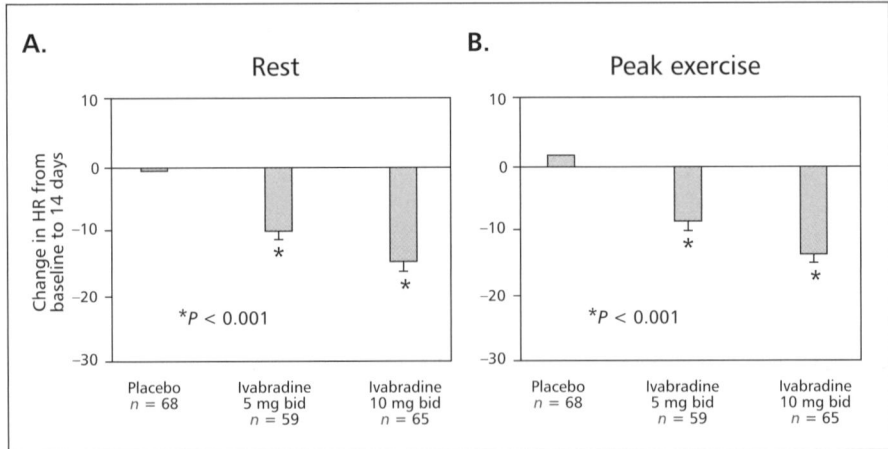

Figure 2 Changes from baseline in heart rate (HR) at rest (A) and at peak of exercise (B) in the different treatment groups, at trough of drug activity at the end of the double-blind, dose-ranging phase. From Borer et al.[21]

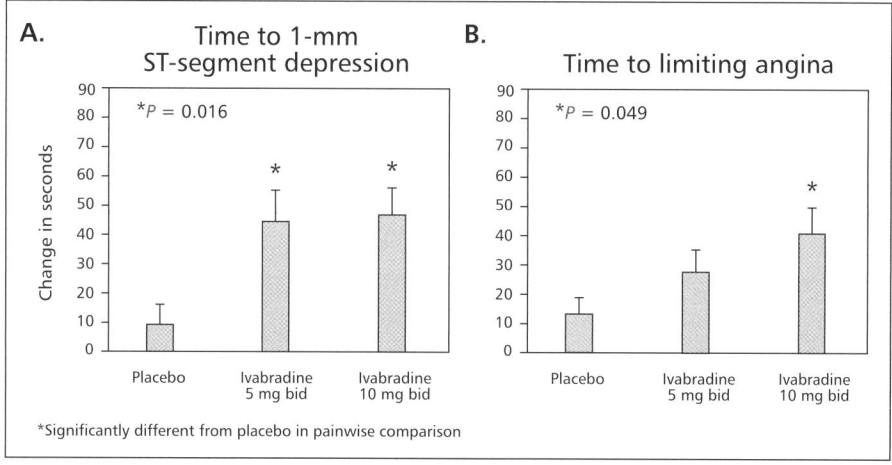

Figure 3 Changes in exercise tolerance test criteria at trough of drug activity during the double-blind, dose-ranging phase. From Borer et al.[21]

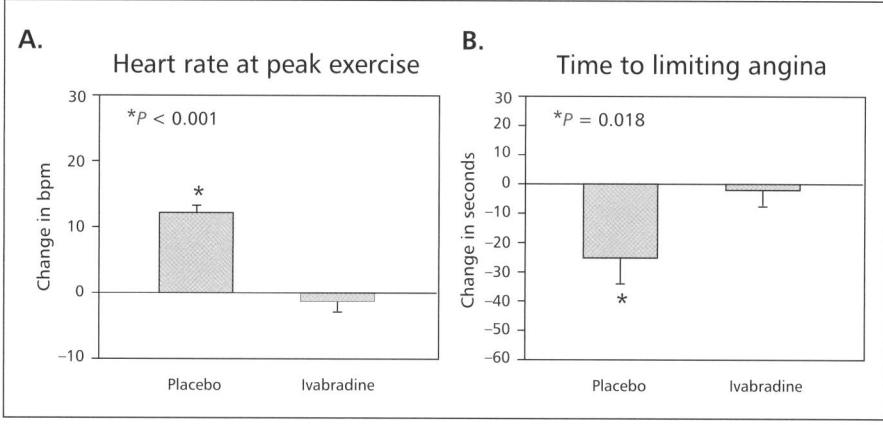

Figure 4 Changes in maximal heart rate and increase in time to limiting angina during the double-blind randomized withdrawal period. Patients withdrawn to placebo had significant deteriorations in exercise test parameters. From Borer et al.[21]

IVABRADINE VERSUS ATENOLOL IN THE INITIATIVE TRIAL

Prompted by these encouraging results, we conducted the larger INITIATIVE trial – a randomized, double-blind, multicenter study in 939 patients with chronic stable angina, involving 144 centers in 21 countries. This study evaluated the anti-anginal and anti-ischemic effects of the I_f inhibitor ivabradine vs. the β-blocker atenolol.[22] The primary objective of the INITIATIVE trial was to confirm that ivabradine was equally as effective as atenolol in improving exercise capacity. Eligibility criteria for patients to enter the study were a history of at least 3 months of chronic stable angina, as well as evidence of underlying coronary artery disease manifested by at least one of the following five criteria: a history of myocardial infarction confirmed by Q wave and/or cardiac enzyme elevation ≥ 3 months before study entry; coronary angioplasty performed ≥ 6 months before study entry; bypass surgery performed ≥ 3 months before study entry; a coronary angiogram showing a diameter stenosis of ≥ 50% in the proximal two-thirds of one or more of the major coronary arteries; or scintigraphic or echocardiographic evidence of exercise-induced, reversible myocardial ischemia.

After placebo wash-out of all anti-anginal medications – over a period of 2–7 days, depending on the previously administered treatment (≥ 5 half-lives) – patients were randomized to one of three treatment groups: ivabradine 5 mg bid for 4 weeks, increasing to 7.5 mg bid for 12 weeks; ivabradine 5 mg bid for 4 weeks, increasing to 10 mg bid for 12 weeks; or atenolol 50 mg od for 4 weeks, increasing to 100 mg od for the following 12 weeks (*Figure 5*).

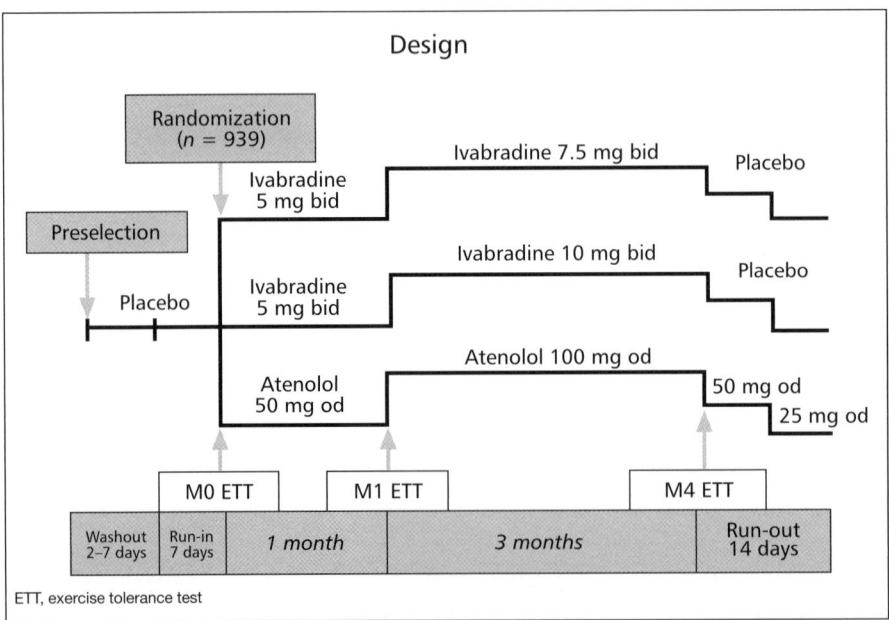

Figure 5 Study design of the INITIATIVE trial

The primary efficacy endpoint was the change from baseline to end of treatment (16 weeks) in total exercise duration during treadmill ETTs performed according to a modified Bruce protocol at trough of drug activity. There was no consensus on the clinical equivalence limit that should define treadmill ETT criteria in non-inferiority trials in patients with stable angina. Taking into account the mean change from baseline in total exercise duration, and the standard deviation of this change estimated by independent statisticians using data observed in a blinded review of the first 200 patients, an equivalence limit of 35 s (i.e. a non-inferiority limit equal to −35 s) was recommended by an independent expert committee. Secondary endpoints included changes in time to limiting angina; time to onset of angina; and time to 1-mm ST-segment depression, both at trough and peak of drug activity. Frequency of angina attack and short-acting nitrate consumption were also evaluated from patients' diaries.

The mean age of patients was 61 years, and more than 80% were men. Approximately 70% of patients had class 2 angina; 54% had a prior history of myocardial infarction; 19% had previously undergone percutaneous coronary interventions; and 18% had undergone coronary artery bypass graft surgery. The total duration of exercise at trough of drug activity (mean ± SD) increased from inclusion to end of treatment (16 weeks of therapy) by 86.8 ± 129.0 s with ivabradine 7.5 mg bid; 91.7 ± 118.8 s with ivabradine 10 mg bid; and 78.8 ± 133.4 s with atenolol 100 mg od. The mean differences, when compared with atenolol 100 mg, were 10.3 ± 9.4 s and 15.7 ± 9.5 s in favor of ivabradine 7.5 and 10 mg ($p < 0.001$ for non-inferiority; *Figure 6*). No significant difference was observed

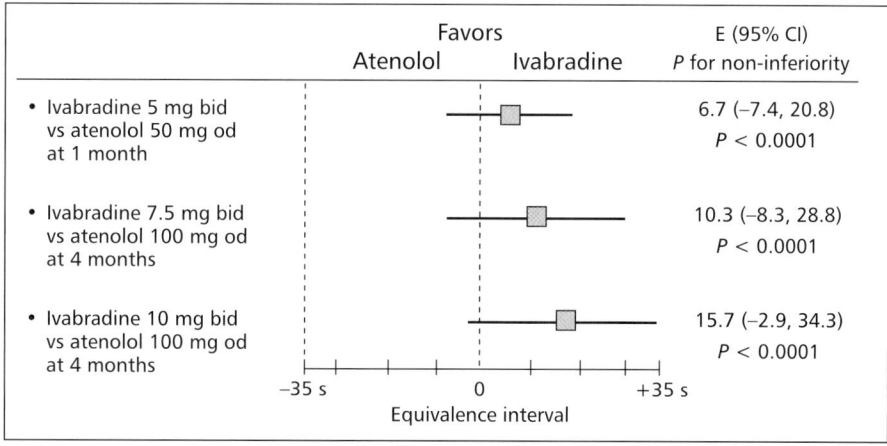

Figure 6 Differences in the change in total exercise duration at trough of drug activity for ivabradine vs. atenolol

between the ivabradine groups, with an adjusted estimated difference of 5.4 s (95% CI: −12.9, 23.8). Time to 1-mm ST-segment depression increased by 98.0 ± 153.7 s with ivabradine 7.5 mg bid; 86.9 ± 128.2 s with ivabradine 10 mg bid; and 95.6 ± 147.5 s with atenolol 100 mg od ($P < 0.001$ and $P = 0.002$ for non-inferiority of ivabradine 7.5 mg and 10 mg vs. atenolol 100 mg, respectively). This increase in time to 1-mm ST-segment depression by approximately 1.5 min with ivabradine indicates that the improvement in total exercise capacity was mediated by a relevant anti-ischemic effect. Total exercise duration after 4 weeks of therapy improved by 64.2 ± 104.0 s with ivabradine 5 mg, and by 60.0 ± 114.4 s with atenolol 50 mg ($P < 0.001$ for non-inferiority). Non-inferiority of ivabradine was demonstrated at all doses and for all criteria, including time to limiting angina, in both the intention-to-treat and per-protocol populations (*Figure* 7).

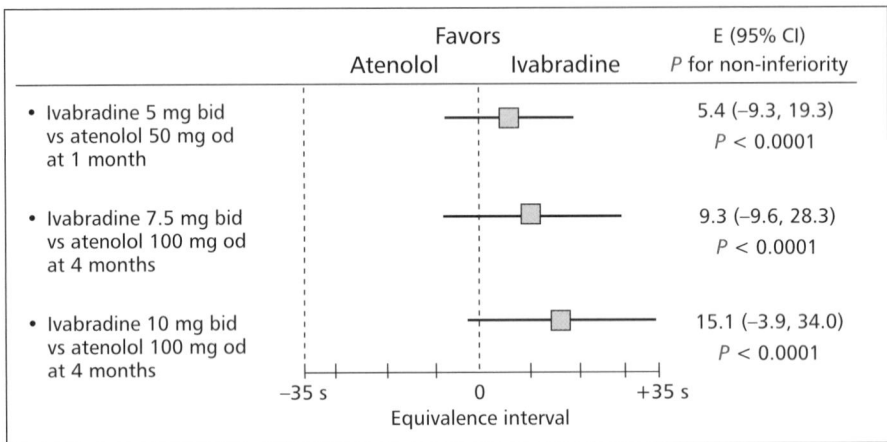

Figure 7 Differences in the change in time to limiting angina at trough of drug activity in the study groups

Heart rate and rate pressure product were reduced at the end of the treatment period, compared with baseline, at rest as well as at peak of exercise. At peak of exercise, the decrease in heart rate was greater in patients treated with atenolol (14.0 bpm) than in those receiving ivabradine 7.5 mg and 10 mg (8.6 bpm and 10.3 bpm, respectively), showing that ivabradine induced a similar or greater improvement in exercise capacity than atenolol for a comparatively lower rate pressure product and heart rate reduction. The number of angina attacks per week was decreased by two-thirds over the 4-month treatment period with both ivabradine and atenolol, to approximately one attack per week. Thus, the

INITIATIVE trial has shown that ivabradine is as effective as atenolol for the treatment of stable angina.[22]

OTHER TRIALS WITH IVABRADINE

The non-inferiority of ivabradine at doses of 7.5 mg bid and 10 mg bid was compared with amlodipine 10 mg od during 3 months of therapy in a randomized clinical trial that involved 1195 patients with chronic stable angina and documented coronary artery disease.[23] Approximately 67% and 18% of patients had class 2 and class 3 angina, respectively. In the study, ivabradine 7.5 mg bid was found to have efficacy indistinguishable from that of amlodipine 10 mg od for all measured bicycle exercise test parameters (*Figure 8*). The total exercise duration was considerably increased at trough of drug activity, by 27.6 s and 21.7 s, respectively, with ivabradine 7.5 mg and 10 mg bid. Time to angina onset and time to 1-mm ST-segment depression were also increased.

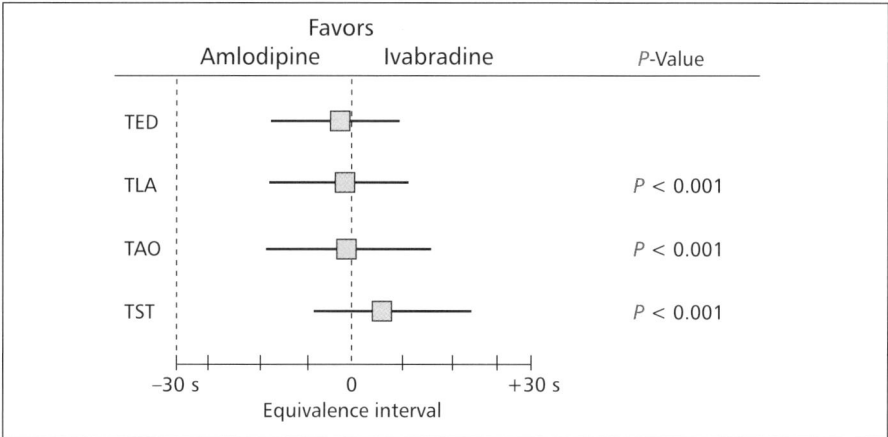

Figure 8 Changes in exercise tolerance test parameters in the ivabradine 7.5 mg bid group and in the amlodipine 10 mg od group. TED, total exercise duration; TLA, time to limiting angina; TAO, time to angina onset; TST, time to 1-mm ST-segment depression

Considerable evidence suggests that combination therapy may be more effective than monotherapy for the treatment of angina pectoris.[1] The efficacy and safety of a combination therapy has been established over a year in 386 patients with stable angina already treated by nitrates or dihydropyridine calcium-channel blockers.[24] Two different dosages of ivabradine were used:

5 mg and 7.5 mg bid. Ivabradine was shown to reduce the heart rate of patients by 10 bpm at 5 mg bid, and 12 bpm at 7.5 mg bid. Ivabradine maintained this heart rate reduction over the year of follow-up. The number of angina attacks reported by patients were significantly reduced.

POTENTIAL ANTI-ATHEROSCLEROTIC EFFECTS OF HEART RATE REDUCTION

The relationship between resting heart rate and cardiovascular events has been documented in numerous epidemiological studies in different populations, including elderly patients and those with hypertension or the metabolic syndrome (see Chapter 1). Experimental data have demonstrated that a reduction in heart rate can delay the progression of coronary and carotid atherosclerosis in animal models.[25,26] This association between heart rate and atherosclerosis has also been observed in humans,[27,28] where disease progression was predicted independently by minimum heart rate in a study of 56 men who had developed myocardial infarction at a young age. Coronary artery endothelial cell dysfunction associated with high heart rates may represent an important mechanism for this increased atherogenesis.[29,30] More recently, positive associations have been identified between plaque disruption, an elevated left-ventricular mass and a mean heart rate > 80 bpm, while a negative association with the use of β-blockers was also demonstrated.[31] These observations are supported by results from the β-blocker Cholesterol-lowering Asymptomatic Plaque Study (BCAPS), which demonstrated a reduction in the rate of progression of carotid intima-media thickness with the use of a β-blocker in asymptomatic patients.[32] In addition to its anti-anginal effects, this may therefore represent a potentially important target for ivabradine.

CONCLUSIONS

Ivabradine is a selective and specific I_f inhibitor with anti-anginal and anti-ischemic effects that have been shown to be non-inferior to those of the β-blocker atenolol and the calcium-channel blocker amlodipine. Unlike β-blockers, ivabradine is devoid of intrinsic negative inotropic effects and does not affect coronary vasomotion. A wide range of patients with angina may benefit from exclusive heart rate reduction with ivabradine, including newly diagnosed stable angina patients, those with contraindications or intolerance to the use of β-blockers, as well as patients who are insufficiently controlled by β-blockers or calcium-channel blockers.

REFERENCES

1. Management of stable angina pectoris. Recommendations of the Task Force of the European Society of Cardiology. *Eur Heart J*. 1997;18:394–413.

2. Guth BD, Heusch G, Seitelberger R, Ross J Jr, et al. Mechanism of beneficial effect of beta-adrenergic blockade on exercise-induced myocardial ischemia in conscious dogs. *Circ Res*. 1987;60:738–746.

3. North of England Stable Angina Guideline Development Group. North of England evidence based guidelines development project: summary version of evidence based guideline for the primary care management of angina. *BMJ*. 1996;312:827–832.

4. Ko DT, Hebert PR, Coffey CS, et al. Beta-blocker therapy and symptoms of depression, fatigue, and sexual dysfunction. *JAMA*. 2002:288:351–357.

5. Fogari R, Zoppi A, Corradi L, et al. Sexual function in hypertensive males treated with lisinopril or atenolol: a cross-over study. *Am J Hypertens*. 1998;11:1244–1247.

6. Tafreshi MJ, Weinacher AB. Beta-adrenergic-blocking agents in bronchospastic diseases: a therapeutic dilemma. *Pharmacotherapy*. 1999;19:974–978.

7. Freytag F, Schelling A, Meinicke T, Deichsel G. Telmisartan Hypertension Experience in a Randomized European Study Versus Atenolol Study Group. Comparison of 26-week efficacy and tolerability of telmisartan and atenolol, in combination with hydrochlorothiazide as required, in the treatment of mild to moderate hypertension: a randomized, multicenter study. *Clin Ther*. 2001;23: 108–123.

8. Bortone AS, Hess OM, Gaglione A, et al. Effect of intravenous propranolol on coronary vasomotion at rest and during dynamic exercise in patients with coronary artery disease. *Circulation*. 1990;81:1225–1235.

9. Berdeaux A, Drieu la Rochelle C, Richard V, Giudicelli JF. Opposed responses of large and small coronary arteries to propranolol during exercise in dogs. *Am J Physiol*. 1991;261:H265–H270.

10. Simon L, Ghaleh B, Puybasset L, et al. Coronary and hemodynamic effects of S 16257, a new bradycardic agent, in resting and exercising conscious dogs. *J Pharmacol Exp Ther*. 1995;275:659–666.

11. Krone W, Nagele H. Effects of antihypertensives on plasma lipids and lipoprotein metabolism. *Am Heart J*. 1988;116:1729–1734.

12. Reneland R, Alvarez E, Andersson PE, et al. Induction of insulin resistance by beta-blockade but not ACE inhibition: long-term treatment with atenolol or trandolapril. *J Hum Hypertens*. 2000;14:175–180.

13. DiFrancesco D. Characterization of single pacemaker channels in cardiac sino-atrial node cells. *Nature*. 1986;324:470–473.

14. DiFrancesco D. The contribution of the "pacemaker" current (If) to generation of spontaneous activity in rabbit sino-atrial node myocytes. *J Physiol*. 1991;434:23–40.

15. Bois P, Bescond J, Renaudon B, et al. Mode of action of bradycardic agent, S 16257, on ionic currents of rabbit sinoatrial node cells. *Br J Pharmacol*. 1996;118:1051–1057.

16. Thollon C, Cambarrat C, Vian J, et al. Electrophysiological effects of S 16257, a novel sino-atrial node modulator, on rabbit and guinea-pig cardiac preparations: comparison with UL–FS 49. *Br J Pharmacol*. 1994;112:37–42.

17. Gardiner SM, Kemp PA, March JE, et al. Acute and chronic cardiac and regional haemodynamic effects of the novel bradycardic agent, S 16257, in conscious rats. *Br J Pharmacol*. 1995;115:579–586.

18. Ragueneau I, Laveille C, Jochemsen R, et al. Pharmacokinetic-pharmacodynamic modeling of the effects of ivabradine, a direct sinus node inhibitor, on heart rate in healthy volunteers. *Clin Pharmacol Ther*. 1998;64:192–203.

19. Bel A, Perrault LP, Faris B, et al. Inhibition of the pacemaker current: a bradycardic therapy for off-pump coronary operations. *Ann Thorac Surg*. 1998;66:148–152.

20. Vilaine JP, et al. Procoralan, a new selective If current inhibitor. *Eur Heart J*. 2003;5(Suppl G):G26–G35.

21. Borer JS, Fox K, Jaillon P, et al. Antianginal and antiischemic effects of ivabradine, an I(f) inhibitor, in stable angina: a randomized, double-blind, multicentered, placebo-controlled trial. *Circulation*. 2003;107:817–823.

22. Tardif J, Ford M, Tendera K. Anti-anginal and anti-ischemic effects of the If current inhibitor ivabradine versus atenolol in stable angina. A 4-month randomised, double-blind, multicenter trial. *Eur Heart J*. 2003;24(Suppl):20.

23. Ruzyllo W, Ford I, Tendera M, et al. Antianginal and antiischaemic effects of the If current inhibitor ivabradine compared to amlodipine as monotherapies in patients with chronic stable angina. Randomized, controlled double blind trial. *Circulation*. 2004;25(Suppl):Abstract 878.

24. Lopez-Bescos L, Filipova S, Martos R, et al. Long-term safety and antianginal efficacy of the If current inhibitor ivabradine in patients with chronic stable angina. A one-year randomized, double blind, multicenter trial. *Circulation*. 2004;25(Suppl):Abstract 876.

25. Beere PA, Glagov S, Zarins CK. Retarding effect of lowered heart rate on coronary atherosclerosis. *Science*. 1984;226:180–182.

26. Tardif JC, Gregoire J, L'Allier PL, Joyal M. Chronic heart reduction with ivabradine and prevention of atherosclerosis progression assessed using intravascular ultrasound. *Eur Heart J*. 2003.

27. Perski A, Hamsten A, Lindvall K, Theorell T. Heart rate correlates with severity of coronary atherosclerosis in young postinfarction patients. *Am Heart J*. 1988;116:1369–1373.

28. Perski A, Olsson G, Landou C, et al. Minimum heart rate and coronary atherosclerosis: independent relations to global severity and rate of progression of angiographic lesions in men with myocardial infarction at a young age. *Am Heart J*. 1992;123:609–616.

29. Strawn WB, Bondjers G, Kaplan JR, et al. Endothelial dysfunction in response to psychosocial stress in monkeys. *Circ Res*. 1991;68:1270–1279.

30. Skantze HB, Kaplan J, Pettersson J, et al. Psychosocial stress causes endothelial injury in cynomolgus monkeys via beta1-adrenoceptor activation. *Atherosclerosis*. 1998;136:153–161.

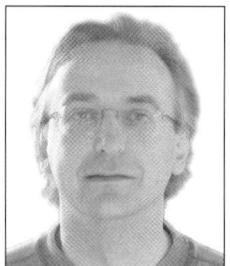

Nicolas Danchin

6 Potential indications for exclusive heart rate reduction for the future

Nicolas Danchin

Hôpital Européen Georges Pompidou
20 Rue Leblanc
75015 Paris, France
Email : nicolas.danchin@egp.ap-hop-paris.fr

Many epidemiologic studies have found strong correlations between resting heart rate and long-term outcomes.[1-3] However, beyond these findings, there are many reasons to believe that heart rate reduction might prove beneficial in coronary artery disease patients. Obviously, the larger part of coronary perfusion takes place during diastole, where wall stress is considerably less than during systole, and the role of a lower heart rate in prolonging the diastolic time is patent. We will describe some of the available evidence linking heart rate with coronary artery disease; we will then review some data on the clinical impact of measures aimed at lowering heart rate on myocardial ischemia, with a special focus on the new class of inhibitors of the I_f current.

ROLE OF HEART RATE IN THE DEVELOPMENT AND CLINICAL COURSE OF CORONARY ARTERY DISEASE

Experimental data suggest a potent link between heart rate and development of coronary artery atherosclerosis. Several experiments in monkeys have shown that increased heart rate was associated with a higher risk of developing coronary artery disease.[4,5] More recently, also in a simian model, it was shown that the animals with the lowest heart rate had less carotid atherosclerosis,[6] while another study showed that the thickness of aortic or iliac plaques was correlated with the rate–pressure product,[7] suggesting that heart rate might impact on the development of coronary as well as extracoronary atherosclerosis.

Beyond the beneficial effect of a lower heart rate in terms of prevention of atherosclerosis, a lower heart rate might also help avoid some of the most dreaded complications of coronary artery disease. In this regard, an elegant angiographic study suggests a possible explanation: a lower heart rate might provide protection against the risk of coronary plaque rupture.[7] In this study, 53 patients having undergone two coronary angiograms 6 months apart and showing evidence of rupture of a smooth atherosclerotic plaque on the second angiogram were matched for age and sex with 53 patients without such signs of plaque rupture. The two best independent predictors of plaque rupture were increased left ventricular mass > 270 g (odds ratio: 4.92, 95% confidence interval: 1.83–13.2) and mean resting heart rate over 24 hours at the time of the first angiogram > 80 beats per minute (odds ratio: 3.19; 95% confidence interval: 1.15–8.85). In addition, treatment with β-blockers was associated with a significant independent reduction in the risk of plaque rupture, while treatment with angiotensin-converting enzyme inhibitors or statins was associated with a strong trend toward a reduction in the risk of plaque rupture ($P = 0.06$).

CLINICAL CONSEQUENCES OF HEART RATE MODIFICATION

Non-pharmacological intervention

Physical training and cardiac rehabilitation can lower heart rate, both at baseline and during exercise, resulting in an increase in exercise capacity. In patients with recent myocardial infarction, β-blocker therapy alone is insufficient to improve exercise duration and maximal workload or decrease the rate–pressure product, while all three parameters improve in patients undergoing physical training, with or without concomitant β-blocker therapy.[8] Recently, the results of a randomized trial comparing physical training and percutaneous coronary interventions in 101 patients with stable coronary artery disease were reported.[9] Patients in the exercise training group first had a 2-week hospital program of physical training, and were then asked to exercise daily. At 2 years of follow-up, resting heart rate was lower in the exercise training group. A similar improvement in the Canadian classification of angina and maximal oxygen consumption during stress testing was observed in the two groups. Event-free survival, however, was higher in the rehabilitation group (88% versus 70%), mainly because there were more reinterventions in the group having undergone coronary angioplasty.

β-Blocking agents

Among medications, the class of anti-ischemic agents with the most important impact on heart rate is obviously that of β-blockers. In the recent past, data have suggested that β-blockers might have additional efficacy, compared with other antianginal medications having similar direct anti-ischemic properties. In a series of 352 patients with stable coronary artery disease having undergone thallium single photon emission computed tomography (SPECT), Marie et al.[10] analyzed the prognostic influence of therapeutic changes immediately after the exercise test. The presence of myocardial ischemia documented by thallium SPECT was a strong predictor of major coronary events in the whole population; in patients who received β-blocking agents after the test, however, the prognostic impact of exercise ischemia disappeared, whereas it remained present in patients who received additional antianginal medications when these medications did not include β-blockers. Whether the additional protection conferred by β-blockers might be partially or totally related to their heart rate-lowering capacity remains speculative. Concordant data, however, suggest that heart rate reduction with β-blockers might be one of the main reasons for their efficacy. After myocardial infarction, β-blocking agents improve long-term prognosis.[11] When β-blockers are classified according to their pharmacologic properties, however, those with an intrinsic sympathomimetic activity appear to be less efficacious than those without intrinsic sympathomimetic activity. Likewise, a very strong correlation is observed between the reduction in mortality with β-blockers and the decrease in heart rate observed in the randomized trials carried out with different β-blocking agents in the post-myocardial infarction setting.[12] In the CIBIS-II trial, which assessed the role of β-blockade with bisoprolol in patients with congestive heart failure,[13] changes in heart rate were recorded in patients alive 2 months after inclusion in the trial and their impact on long-term survival was assessed. Using multivariate analyses, both a lower baseline heart rate and a higher degree of heart rate reduction during the first 2 months were independently correlated with late mortality. In patients with sinus rhythm at baseline, treatment with bisoprolol was an additional predictor of improved survival, independently of baseline heart rate and of heart rate reduction, suggesting independent roles for heart rate reduction and use of the β-blocking agent bisoprolol in this setting.

I_f current inhibitors: clinical data

I_f current inhibitors have the unique property of reducing heart rate without having any hemodynamic impact. The first I_f current inhibitor tested in the clinical setting of stable coronary artery disease was zatebradine. In a dose-finding trial comparing its antianginal efficacy with placebo, it was found that, at peak activity of the highest dose used (7.5 mg bid), zatebradine significantly increased the time to 1-mm ST-segment depression, with a trend to a longer total exercise duration.[15] The clinical development of zatebradine, however, was not pursued.

Ivabradine is a selective I_f current inhibitor with no effect on the QT interval in experimental studies. A pivotal multicenter randomized trial comparing 3 dosages of ivabradine with placebo in patients with stable coronary artery disease was recently published;[16] 360 patients were randomized according to a double-blind technique to either placebo, or ivabradine 2.5 mg, 5 mg or 10 mg twice a day for 2 weeks. The primary end points of the trial were the evolution in time to limiting angina and time to 1-mm ST-segment depression at the trough of the study medication. Following this double-blind period, 170 patients were included in an open-label ivabradine (10 mg bid) phase for 2 to 3 months, depending on administrative requirements in the different participating countries. After this open-label phase, the patients were again randomized to a 1-week double-blind runout phase between placebo or continued ivabradine. Heart rate at rest as well as at peak exercise decreased in a dose-dependent manner with ivabradine. Time to 1-mm ST-segment depression increased by 46 seconds in the 10 mg bid ivabradine group, compared with 9 seconds in the placebo group (*Figure 1*).

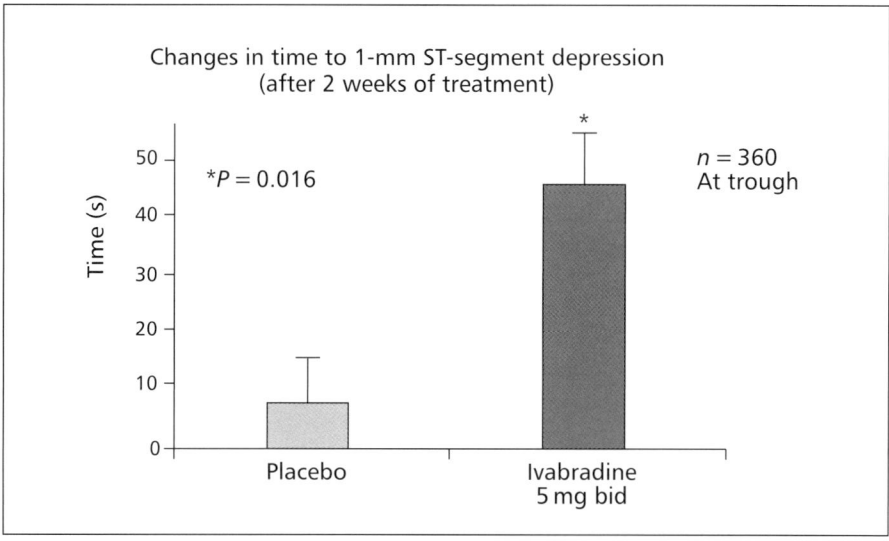

Figure 1 At trough of drug activity, ivabradine significantly increases time to 1-mm ST-segment depression

Likewise, time to limiting angina increased in a dose-dependent manner with increasing doses of ivabradine. During the open-label phase all parameters increased in the groups which were not previously receiving the highest dose of ivabradine. Finally, during the runout phase, no rebound effect was noted after the interruption of ivabradine.

Two other trials were presented in part during the 2003 meeting of the European Society of Cardiology. Both trials were designed as non-inferiority trials. The trial versus amlodipine included 1195 patients and compared two dosages of ivabradine (7.5 mg bid and 10 mg bid) with amlodipine 10 mg od. At the 7.5 mg bid dose, ivabradine was non-inferior to amlodipine for all exercise testing parameters. The trial versus atenolol included 939 patients; in a first phase of 1 month's duration, atenolol 50 mg od was compared with ivabradine 5 mg bid;

during the second, 3-month duration phase, doses were increased to 100 mg od for atenolol, 7.5 mg bid and 10 mg bid for ivabradine. With respect to the time to limiting angina at trough, ivabradine 5 mg bid was not inferior to atenolol 50 mg od, and ivabradine 7.5 mg bid and 10 mg bid were not inferior to atenolol 100 mg od. (*Figure 2*)

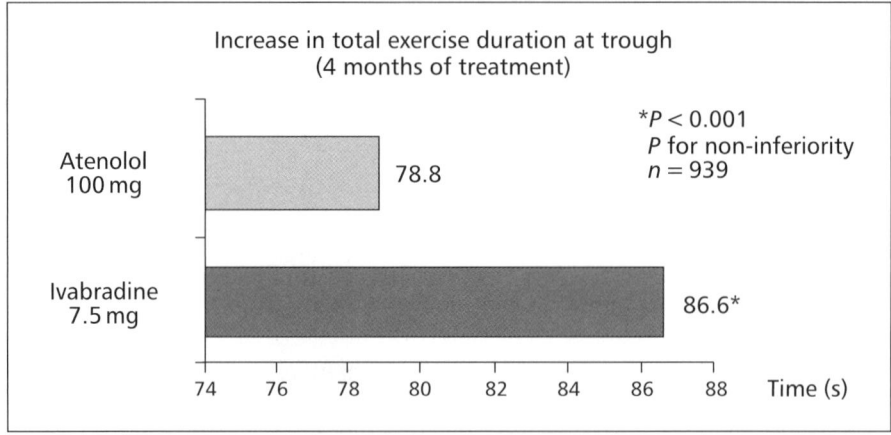

Figure 2 Ivabradine increases total exercise duration, at trough of drug activity

Overall these studies confirm that heart rate reduction alone can limit exercise-induced myocardial ischemia.

Many patients with coronary artery disease do not receive β-blockers

In spite of all the evidence leading to the recommendations regarding the use of β-blockers in patients with myocardial infarction, all observational studies show that many patients are not prescribed β-blocking agents after acute coronary syndromes.[17,18] Though some of these patients have authentic contraindications, many are not prescribed these agents mainly because of the reluctance of the physicians to use these medications, which are perceived as having too many potentially severe side-effects (*Figure 3*).[19]

These include a definite risk of bronchospasm, and a risk of acute heart failure when the medication is initiated in patients with poor left ventricular function. Heart rate-lowering agents which do not have such side-effects might therefore be easier to prescribe, and could be used in patients in whom β-blockers are not prescribed.

Effect	Comment
• Bradycardia	• Absolute contraindication in 2nd and 3rd degree heart block. Caution with other heart rate-lowering agents
• Hypotension	• May be exacerbated when used with potent vasodilators
• Reduced contractility (negative inotropism)	• Because of myocardial depression, initiate with caution in stable heart failure. Avoid in worsening unstable heart failure
• Bronchospasm	• May precipitate (life-threatening) asthma. Avoid in those with history of asthma or COAD, or use cardioselective agent with extreme (supervised) caution
• Cold extremities	• May be less common in agents with partial agonism. Avoid in Raynaud's disease
• Lethargy/fatigue	• May adversely affect compliance
• Nightmares/sleep disturbances	• May relate to lipophilicity. Possibly reduced with hydrophilic agents, e.g., atenolol
• Inhibition of metabolic/ autonomic responses to hypoglycemia	• May mask symptoms of hypoglycemia in insulin-treated diabetics. Avoid in those with frequent hypoglycemia or taking sulfonylureas
• Impotence/reduced sexual activity	• Likely to be more common with β-blockers used with thiazide diuretics. Generally not commonly reported in monotherapy trials

Figure 3 Effects that may limit or contraindicate use of β-blocker drugs. COAD, chronic obstructive airways disease. Reproduced by permission of Laboratoires Servier

Heart rate reduction with I_f current inhibitors: further perspectives in coronary artery disease – acute heart failure and diastolic heart failure

I_f current inhibitors have the unique property of decreasing heart rate without depressing left ventricular function. In acute situations, such as the acute stage of myocardial infarction, a high heart rate on admission is a strong correlate of mortality. In a prospective registry of patients admitted for acute myocardial infarction in France in 2000, heart rate > 90 beats per minute on admission was associated with a 76% increase in the risk of in-hospital mortality after multivariate adjustment.[17] In such situations, the capacity to decrease heart rate without altering cardiac contractility would appear particularly useful. In addition, in the case of acute heart failure complicating acute myocardial infarction, the use of sympathomimetic agents such as dobutamine or dopamine is usually warranted. However, in clinical practice, the increase in heart rate caused by dobutamine often constitutes a limitation for its use, particularly at high dosages. The combined use of heart rate-controlling medications might prove particularly helpful, provided these medications do not cause any additional impairment in left ventricular function. There is experimental evidence, in a rat model of myocardial stunning caused by a sequence of ischemia–reperfusion, that the concomitant use of dobutamine and ivabradine permits avoidance of the tachycardia generated by dobutamine, without impairing mean arterial pressure, or the recovery of left ventricular wall thickening and left ventricular fractional shortening achieved with dobutamine (V. Richard, personal communication).

With the constant aging of patient populations in industrialized countries, diastolic heart failure represents an increasingly frequent cause of cardiac failure. The therapeutic management of these patients is complex, as only very few patients with diastolic heart failure were enrolled in the large randomized trials in heart failure. As stated by the Task Force of the European Society of Cardiology for the diagnosis and treatment of chronic heart failure,[20] therapeutic recommendations therefore remain largely speculative. Nevertheless, because of the pathophysiologic mechanisms of diastolic dysfunction, medications that improve relaxation by reducing heart rate and increasing the diastolic period are recommended: to date, these medications were mainly represented by β-blockers and verapamil-type calcium antagonists, which were recommended as first-line therapy by the European Task Force. Ivabradine, by its ability to prolong the diastolic period without impairing ventricular contractility, might be particularly helpful in the specific setting of diastolic heart failure. Colin et al.[21] examined left ventricular relaxation in response to saline infusion, atenolol, or ivabradine in dogs at rest and during exercise. Under saline, heart rate increased from 108 to 220 beats per minute, and the relaxation constant τ_{BF} decreased from 22 to 14 ms. Both atenolol and ivabradine significantly limited the increase in heart rate during exercise to about 150 beats per minute. Concomitantly, atenolol prevented the decrease in τ_{BF} (23 ms), while ivabradine did not (15 ms). In brief, ivabradine limited exercise-induced tachycardia, without simultaneously altering the exercise-induced acceleration of the rate of left ventricular relaxation; in contrast, for the same levels of limitation of heart rate during exercise, atenolol did prevent the acceleration of the rate of ventricular relaxation. Therefore, ivabradine, which can preserve left ventricular relaxation even during exercise, might prove particularly beneficial in patients with diastolic heart failure.

CONCLUSION

There is ample evidence of an association between high heart rate and poor outcome in numerous clinical settings. The concept of a causal relationship between higher heart rate and poorer cardiovascular outcomes is reinforced by the fact that β-blockers have a well-documented efficacy in secondary prevention after myocardial infarction, although the other properties of these agents may also participate in their protective effect. Medications capable of decreasing heart rate without affecting left ventricular function might be especially valuable, particularly in patients with contraindications to β-blockers, or in patients with acute heart failure.

REFERENCES

1.   Dyer AR, Persky V, Stamler J, et al. Heart rate as a prognostic factor for coronary heart disease and mortality: findings in three Chicago epidemiologic studies. *Am J Epidemiol*. 1980;112:736–749.

2.   Hjalmarson A, Gilpin EA, Kjekshus J, et al. Influence of heart rate on mortality after myocardial infarction. *Am J Cardiol*. 1990;65:547–553.

3.   Aronow WS, Ahn C, Mercando AD, Epstein S. Association of average heart rate on 24-hour ambulatory electrocardiograms with incidence of new coronary events at 48-month follow-up in 1,311 patients (mean age 81 years) with heart disease and sinus rhythm. *Am J Cardiol*. 1996;78:1175–1176.

4.   Beere PA, Glagov S, Zarins CK. Retarding effect of lowered heart rate on coronary atherosclerosis. *Science*. 1984;226:180–182.

5.   Kaplan JR, Manuck SB, Clarkson TB. The influence of heart rate on coronary atherosclerosis. *J Cardiovasc Pharmacol*. 1987;10(Suppl. 2):S100–S102.

6.   Beere PA, Glagov S, Zarins CK. Experimental atherosclerosis at the carotid bifurcation of the cynomolgus monkey. Localization, compensatory enlargement, and the sparing effect of lowered heart rate. *Arterioscler Thromb*. 1992;12: 1245–1253.

7.   Heidland UE, Strauer BE. Left ventricular muscle mass and elevated heart rate are associated with coronary plaque disruption. *Circulation*. 2001;104:1477–1482.

8.   Malfatto G, Facchini M, Sala L, et al. Effects of cardiac rehabilitation and beta-blocker therapy on heart rate variability after first acute myocardial infarction. *Am J Cardiol*. 1998;81:834–840.

9. Hambrecht R, Walther C, Möbius-Winckler S, et al. Percutaneous coronary angioplasty compared with exercise training in patients with stable coronary artery disease. A randomized trial. *Circulation*. 2004;109:1371–1378.

10. Marie PY, Danchin N, Branly F, et al. Effects of medical therapy on outcome assessment using exercise thallium-201 single photon emission computed tomography imaging. Evidence of a protective effect of beta-blocking antianginal medications. *J Am Coll Cardiol*. 1999;34:113–121.

11. Freemantle N, Cleland J, Young P, Mason J, Harrison J. Beta-blockade after myocardial infarction: systematic review and meta-regression analysis. *BMJ*. 1999;318:1730–1737.

12. Singh BN. Morbidity and mortality in cardiovascular disorders: impact of reduced heart rate. *J Cardiovasc Pharmacol Therapeut*. 2001;6:313–331.

13. Lechat P, Hulot JS, Escolano S, et al. Heart rate and cardiac rhythm relationships with bisoprolol benefit in chronic heart failure in CIBIS II trial. *Circulation*. 2001;103:1428–1433.

14. Aupetit JF, Frassati D, Bui-Xuan B, et al. Efficacy of a beta-adrenergic receptor antagonist, propranolol, in preventing ischaemic ventricular fibrillation: dependence on heart rate and ischaemia duration. *Cardiovasc Res*. 1998;37:646–655.

15. Glasser SP, Michie DD, Thadani U, Baiker WM. Effects of zatebradine (ULFS 49 CL), a sinus node inhibitor, on heart rate and exercise duration in chronic stable angina pectoris. Zatebradine Investigators. *Am J Cardiol*. 1997;79:1401–1405.

16. Borer JS, Fox K, Jaillon P, Lerebours G. Antianginal and anti-ischemic effects of ivabradine, an I_f inhibitor, in stable angina: a randomized, double-blind, multicentered, placebo-controlled trial. *Circulation*. 2003;107:817–823.

17. Hanania G, Cambou JP, Guéret P, et al. Management and in-hospital outcome of patients with acute myocardial infarction admitted to intensive care units at the turn of the century: results from the French nation-wide USIC 2000 registry. *Heart*. 2004;90:1404–1410.

18. Danchin N, Grenier O, Ferrières J, et al. Use of secondary preventive drugs in patients with acute coronary syndromes treated medically or with coronary angioplasty: results from the nationwide French PREVENIR survey. *Heart*. 2002;88 :159–162.

19. Remme WJ, Swedberg K. Task Force for the diagnosis and treatment of chronic heart failure, European Society of Cardiology. Guidelines for the diagnosis and treatment of chronic heart failure. *Eur Heart J*. 2001;22:1527–1560.

20. Purcell H, Fox K. Selective and specific I_f inhibition: New perspectives. *Medicographia*. 2005;27:51–55.

21. Colin P, Ghaleh B, Hittinger L, et al. Differential effects of heart rate reduction and β-blockade on left ventricular relaxation during exercise. *Am J Physiol Heart Circ Physiol*. 2002;282:H672–H679.

Index